1

ISBN: 9781099425516

# WEIGHT MAINTENANCE
## U.S. Edition

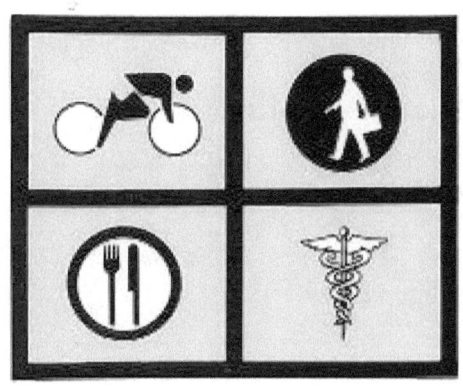

## Vincent Antonetti, Ph.D.

**NoPaperPress**™

# CONTENTS

**10-DAY MINI-DIET**

**LIST OF TABLES**

To millions of people losing weight has become not only a goal but almost a way of life. But researchers have found that most people can lose weight on almost any diet. The crucial concern is whether the weight loss can be maintained. The real challenge is not getting people to lose weight but helping them keep it off. Few, if any, weight control programs have been successful at helping people maintain their weight over the long term. To this writer's knowledge, this eBook is unique in that addresses the two key issues in weight maintenance:

1) **Prevent the regaining of lost weight.**
2) **Prevent weight gain as people age.**

Before we begin, however, some background information.

## Why You Gain Weight After Dieting

After any diet, your lower body weight requires fewer calories to function. In other words, your lower body weight results in a slower metabolism. Within five years, most dieters regain every pound they have lost. Why? In most cases it's because after losing weight most people eventually revert to their pre-diet eating and exercising habits, and this inevitably leads to their regaining the weight they lost – and often more. The fact is the less you weigh, the less you need to eat to maintain your lower weight.

Without some lifestyle modifications, if you are like the average adult you will regain every pound you have lost. It's a fact that 95 percent of dieters gain all the weight they lost back and often more!

## Why You Gain Weight With Age

A study, published in the Annals of Internal Medicine, that followed 4,000 people for three decades suggests that in the long term, 90 percent of men and 70 percent of women will become overweight (with a BMI $\geq$ 25). Interestingly, half of the men and women in the study, who had made it well into adulthood without a weight problem, ultimately also became overweight and a third became obese (with a BMI $\geq$ 30).

Why does this happen? When you reach your mid to late twenties, you slowly start to lose muscle and add fat as part of the natural aging process. As you age your muscle mass slowly deteriorates and is replaced by fat. But muscle is active tissue and requires lots of energy (calories) for growth and repair; whereas, fat is basically inactive and uses very few calories to subsist. So as you age and you lose muscle mass your metabolism gradually slows. In fact, your metabolism decreases about 10 percent every decade. For the average adult, the result of a slowing metabolism is a weight gain of almost 2 pounds every year. To offset this, you need to cut back on the calories you consume, or increase your exercise, or both, or the excess calories will add up and so will your weight! The point being that you can never become complacent. You must continually watch your weight because we are all at risk of becoming overweight.

## Unsuccessful Maintainers
A study published in the American Journal of Preventive Medicine, surveyed approximately 1,300 adults from the 1999 to 2002 who were overweight or obese and lost at least 10 percent of their maximum weight. The study authors found some common factors associated with those who regained their weight:
**1)** They spent four hours or more per day in front of a TV or computer.
**2)** They lost a lot of weight (at least 20 percent of their maximum weight) in a short time.
**3)** They started to regain weight soon after they stopped dieting.
Most of the above make sense. Too much TV or computer time usually means these people are probably getting very little exercise.

It takes time to establish a new lifestyle that supports weight maintenance. People who have lost weight quickly, may not have had the time to acquire all the skills needed to maintain their lower weight.

Losing weight too fast, either by fad or extreme dieting, can leave people feeling deprived and often ends up triggering binges that go on until the lost weight is regained.

## Successful Maintainers
The National Weight Control Registry studied people who had lost at least 30 pounds and kept it off for more than a year. They found that **although people lost weight differently, they kept it off similarly**. Here are some characteristics of the successful maintainers:
**1)** Most eat a moderately low-fat diet.
**2)** Successful maintainers monitor portion sizes.
**3)** Most eat breakfast every day.
**4)** Most are physically active, with walking their most common exercise and they walk for nearly an hour every day. (And these people probably aren't watching TV for four hours daily.)
**5)** Most find pleasure in their healthier lifestyle and diet-free living.

# Knowledge is Power

Health professionals agree that weight maintenance requires a multifaceted approach that includes setting reasonable weight goals, changing eating habits, and getting adequate exercise.

There's no doubt that weight maintenance requires a long-term commitment, and that long-term success is about developing both an understanding and a plan that will result in healthier eating and exercise habits. In brief, the key to successful weight maintenance is lasting lifestyle changes.

Desire and the discipline to start and stay on a weight-maintenance program are crucial. But along with desire and discipline, it is our belief that **only a real understanding of nutrition, exercise and weight control will lead to long-term success**. As is true with many important and complex subjects, to achieve you need more than rules – you need information and a solid understanding. So take the time to read what follows. The reward will last you a lifetime.

Before we begin you should know: What you should weigh? How fit are you? And are you eating properly?

## What Should You Weigh?

Most people want to know what their body weight should be. In 1943, the Metropolitan Life Insurance Company introduced Weight versus Height tables for men and women. (MetLife published revised Weight versus Height tables in 1983.) The tables list weights associated with people who had the lowest mortality rates (lived the longest). The Met Life table yields reasonable weights for women who are slightly shorter than the average height, but the listed weights are not applicable to very short people, and the table lists impossibly low weights for tall women. The tables were also intended for adults ages 25 to 59 years. Their applicability to younger and older adults is problematic. And the MetLife tables would not be appropriate for competitive athletes, body builders, women who are pregnant or breast-feeding and the chronically ill.

More recently, many health-care practitioners rely on Body Mass Index, or BMI, to determine if a person is overweight. The BMI takes into account both a person's weight and height and is calculated by dividing a person's weight in kilograms by the square of their height (in meters). For United States readers, Table 1 provides a convenient way to determine BMI, using body weight in pounds and height in feet and inches. Again, this table would not be applicable to competitive athletes, body builders, women who are pregnant or breast-feeding and the chronically ill.

| Weight (lbs.) | - Height - | | | | | | | | | |
|---|---|---|---|---|---|---|---|---|---|---|
| | 60" | 62" | 64" | 66" | 68" | 70" | 72" | 74" | 76" | 78" |
| 100 | 19.6 | 18.3 | | | | | | | | |
| 110 | 21.5 | 20.1 | 18.9 | 17.8 | | | | | | |
| 120 | 23.5 | 22.0 | 20.6 | 19.4 | 18.3 | | | | | |
| 140 | 27.4 | 25.6 | 24.0 | 22.6 | 21.3 | 20.1 | 19.0 | | | |
| 160 | 31.3 | 29.3 | 27.5 | 25.8 | 24.3 | 23.0 | 21.7 | 20.6 | 19.5 | |
| 180 | 35.2 | 33.0 | 30.9 | 29.0 | 27.4 | 25.8 | 24.4 | 23.1 | 21.9 | 20.8 |
| 200 | 39.1 | 36.6 | 34.3 | 32.3 | 30.4 | 28.7 | 27.1 | 25.7 | 24.3 | 23.1 |
| 220 | 43.0 | 40.3 | 37.8 | 35.5 | 33.4 | 31.3 | 29.8 | 28.2 | 26.8 | 25.4 |
| 240 | 46.9 | 43.9 | 41.2 | 38.7 | 36.5 | 34.4 | 32.6 | 30.8 | 29.2 | 27.8 |
| 260 | 50.8 | 47.6 | 44.7 | 42.0 | 39.5 | 37.3 | 35.3 | 33.4 | 31.6 | 30.1 |
| 280 | | 51.3 | 48.1 | 45.2 | 42.6 | 40.2 | 38.0 | 35.9 | 34.1 | 32.4 |
| 300 | | | 51.5 | 48.5 | 45.6 | 43.0 | 40.7 | 38.6 | 36.5 | 34.7 |
| 400 | | | | | | | 54.3 | 51.4 | 48.7 | 46.3 |

Table 1  Body Mass Index (BMI)

| BMI | Weight Profile |
|---|---|
| 18.5 or less | Underweight |
| 18.6 to 24.9 | Normal |
| 25.0 to 29.9 | Overweight |
| 30.0 to 39.9 | Obese |
| 40 or more | Extremely Obese |

Table 2  Weight Profile vs. BMI

The rationale behind the BMI is based on epidemiological data that show an increase in mortality when the BMI is above 25, although the increase in mortality tends to be moderate until a BMI of 30 is reached.  Table 2 shows how a person's body-weight is categorized as a function of BMI.

## BMI-Based Weight vs. Height

Another more convenient way to use BMI is the **New** BMI-Based Weight vs. Height Chart shown in Table 3, where the normal weight category corresponds to BMI = 18.6 to 24.9, overweight is for BMI = 25.0 to 29.9 and obese is for BMI = 30.0 to 39.9. Not shown in Table 3 is the underweight category (BMI lower than 18.6) and the extremely obese category (BMI greater than 39.9).

### Table 3  BMI-Based Weight vs. Height

| Height | Normal | Overweight | Obese |
|--------|--------|------------|-------|
| 4' 10" | 90 – 119 | 120 – 142 | 143 – 191 |
| 4' 11" | 93 – 123 | 124 – 148 | 149 – 197 |
| 5' 0" | 96 – 127 | 128 – 152 | 153 – 204 |
| 5' 1" | 99 – 131 | 132 – 158 | 159 – 211 |
| 5' 2" | 102 – 135 | 136 – 163 | 164 – 218 |
| 5' 3" | 105 – 140 | 141 – 169 | 170 – 225 |
| 5' 4" | 109 – 144 | 145 – 173 | 174 – 232 |
| 5' 5" | 112 – 149 | 150 – 180 | 181 – 239 |
| 5' 6" | 116 – 154 | 155 – 185 | 186 – 247 |
| 5' 7" | 119 – 159 | 160 – 191 | 192 – 254 |
| 5' 8" | 123 – 163 | 164 – 196 | 197 – 262 |
| 5' 9" | 126 – 168 | 169 – 202 | 203–270 |
| 5' 10" | 130 – 173 | 174 – 206 | 207 – 278 |
| 5' 11" | 134 – 178 | 179 – 214 | 215 – 286 |
| 6' 0" | 137 – 183 | 184 – 220 | 221 – 294 |
| 6' 1" | 141 – 188 | 189 – 227 | 228 – 302 |
| 6' 2" | 145 – 194 | 195 – 232 | 233 – 310 |
| 6' 3" | 149 – 199 | 200 – 239 | 240 – 319 |
| 6' 4" | 152 – 205 | 206 - 246 | 247 - 328 |
| 6' 5" | 157 - 210 | 211 - 252 | 253 – 337 |
| 6' 6" | 161 - 216 | 217 - 259 | 260 - 346 |

**Table 3  BMI-Based Weight vs. Height**

**Example**: Determine BMI of a 5' 6" woman who weighs 160 pounds. First use Table 1. Scan the far left of the table and locate her weight of 160 pounds. From this number run your finger horizontally (to the right) until it intersects the vertical column headed by her 5' 6" (66") height. The number at the intersection is her BMI = 25.8. According to Table 2 she is slightly overweight.

**Example**: Determine the "normal" (healthy) weight range for a 5' 6" woman. From Table 3, find that at 5' 6" she must weigh between 116 and 154 pounds for her weight to be in the "normal" range, that is for her BMI to be between 18.6 and 24.9. (I think you will agree that the normal weight range provided by Table 3 is more useful than the BMI given by Table 1.)

## Waist to Hip Ratio

Another very important weight-profile parameter is your waist-to-hip ratio. Health risks for heart attack and stroke increase considerably for men with a ratio above 1.0 and for women with a ratio above 0.8.

To calculate your waist to hip ratio, measure your waist size (at its narrowest circumference) and divide it by your hip size (at the widest section).

# EXERCISE FUNDAMENTALS

Most successful maintainers get some form of exercise every day. But before you start an exercise regimen you should know your health and fitness status.

## How Fit Are You?

A good measure of your cardio-respiratory fitness, is the volume of oxygen per minute per kilogram of body weight (called $VO_{2max}$) a person can process during hard exercise. Higher values of $VO_{2max}$ indicate better aerobic fitness. For example, a 25 year-old man in excellent physical condition can process about 50 milliliters of oxygen per minute per kilogram of body weight; compared to less than 20 mL/min/kg for a 70 year-old woman in poor condition.

One of the best self assessment tests for $VO_{2max}$ is the Rockport Walking Test. This is a field test, not a laboratory test, and consists of walking one mile as rapidly as you can. At the end of the test you record your pulse and the time it took to complete the walk. You then convert the time to completion and your pulse into $VO_{2max}$ using the formulae. Lastly, you enter Table 1 with your calculated $VO_{2max}$ and determine your cardio-respiratory fitness level.

There is some risk if you take the Rockport Fitness Walking Test without prior conditioning. That is why the following precautions are strongly suggested.
**1)** Be sure to have a medical exam before taking the walking test.
**2)** You should postpone the walking test until you have been exercising regularly for at least one month.
**3)** You must be able to comfortably walk at least two miles before you take the walking test.
When you take the test, if you feel exhausted, experience shortness of breath, become dizzy or light headed, or nauseous, stop the test. Do not attempt a retest until you have exercised regularly for at least another three months, when your fitness level should have improved.

## One-Mile Walking Test

Note: Everyone should **have a medical assessment, or exam**, before starting any weight control and/or physical fitness program. Why? You need to make sure your health status will allow you to modify your caloric intake and increase your physical activity. The medical checkup may be as simple as a visit to a physician who is familiar with your medical history, or it may be a thorough physical exam. Note, in all cases the physician conducting the medical exam should be made aware of and should approve the specific weight management and/or physical fitness program you're planning.

If available, walk on a school track or a measured and marked flat trail with a smooth surface. (Find an old one-quarter mile track and walk four laps on the inside lane for the one-mile test.) You also can use a treadmill rather than a track. Although not as accurate, if need be you can walk a street course you have driven and measured.

Before you start the test, warm up for several minutes with easy walking and stretching. Rest for about one minute. Then start the test. Walk as briskly as possible for one mile, but remember you'll probably walk at least 12 minutes, so don't start too fast. If you still feel strong, pick up the pace on the last lap.

When you finish the test, it's important to immediately measure your pulse. (See page 27 for recommended pulse measurement techniques.) At the conclusion of the test, you should feel slightly winded, but you should not be gasping for air. Your goal is to end the test feeling tired but not exhausted. Remember to cool down by continuing to walk slowly.

| | Age | Cardio-Respiratory Fitness Level | | | |
| --- | --- | --- | --- | --- | --- |
| | | Poor | Fair | Good | Excellent |
| | 20-29 | 33.0-36.4 | 36.5-42.4 | 42.5-46.4 | 46.5-52.4 |
| | 30-39 | 31.5-35.4 | 35.5-40.9 | 41.0-44.9 | 45.0-49.4 |
| Men | 40-49 | 30.2-33.5 | 33.6-38.9 | 39.0-43.7 | 43.8-48.0 |
| | 50-59 | 26.1-30.9 | 31.0-35.7 | 35.8-40.9 | 41.0-45.3 |
| | 60-69 | 20.5-26.0 | 26.1-32.2 | 32.3-36.4 | 36.5-44.2 |
| | 70+ | – No data – | | | |
| | 20-29 | 23.6-28.9 | 29.0-32.9 | 33.0-36.9 | 37.0-41.0 |
| | 30-39 | 22.8-26.9 | 27.0-31.4 | 31.5-35.6 | 35.7-40.0 |
| Women | 40-49 | 21.0-24.4 | 24.5-28.9 | 29.0-32.8 | 32.9-36.9 |
| | 50-59 | 20.2-22.7 | 22.8-26.9 | 27.0-31.4 | 31.5-35.7 |
| | 60-69 | 17.5-20.1 | 20.2-24.4 | 24.5-30.2 | 30.3-31.4 |
| | 70+ | – No data – | | | |

**Table 4: $VO_{2max}$ versus Fitness Level**

**Calculating VO$_{2max}$:** The following is undoubtedly the most difficult portion of this book, because VO$_{2max}$ is a function of so many variables: gender, weight, age, heart rate and time to complete the one-mile test walk. Although the formulae are relatively complex, we have tried to simplify the calculation as much as possible.

For women: VO$_{2max}$ = 133 – W – H – A – T

For men: VO$_{2max}$ = 139 – W – H – A – T, where

W = 0.077 × Weight

A = 0.39 × Age

H = 0.157 × Heart rate

T = 3.26 × Time for mile

**Example:** Determine VO$_{2max}$ and the fitness level of a 29 year-old woman who weighs 150 pounds. She finished the one-mile walking test in 14 minutes and 30 seconds (which is 14.5 minutes) with a heart rate of 145 beats per minute. The first step is to determine values for W, H, A and T.

W = 0.077 × Weight = 0.077 × 150 lbs = 11.6

H = 0.157 × Heart rate = 0.157 × 145 = 22.8

A = 0.39 × Age = 0.39 × 29 years = 11.3

T = 3.26 × Time = 3.26 × 14.5 minutes = 50.5

Then calculate VO$_{2max}$ = 133 – W – H – A – T

VO$_{2max}$ = 133 – 11.6 – 22.8 – 11.3 – 50.5 = 36.8

Finally, enter Table 4 and find that a 29 year-old woman with VO$_{2max}$ = 36.8, her fitness level is good – actually very good bordering on excellent.

## Be More Active Every Day

Before we address exercise programs, here are some ways you can increase physical activity in your daily routine:

Change your attitude toward the occasional "bothersome" physical tasks that you encounter in daily living. Consider anytime you have to lift, bend, reach, walk, as an opportunity to burn additional calories and as an extension of your formal workout.

Look for opportunities to walk, such as walking up stairs (two at a time if you can) rather than using an elevator, walking to a local store rather than driving, walking the course if you play golf, and mowing your lawn. At work stand up and stretch two or three times a day, read standing up, etc.

Engage in leisure activities such as dancing, bowling and gardening more often. They can be enjoyable and provide added exercise.

Each of these daily activities taken alone may not seem like much, but done every day for many years they can add up to a substantial number of extra calories burned.

## Calories Burned

Table 5, on page 17, shows the number of calories burned per hour for various activities. Although the data in the table are from reliable sources, you may find that some of the values are slightly different than those in other books. More important, notice that the calories expended for a given activity depends on your weight. Good news: **For any activity, the more you weigh the more calories you burn!**

**Example**: Determine the number of calories burned by a 187-pound woman (or man) who walks seven miles in two hours.

First calculate the person's walking speed = 7 miles / 2 hours = 3.5 mph. Because 187 lbs is not listed in Table 5 (page 17), we use the neighboring weight of 180 lbs. Then from Table 5 we find that walking at 3.5 mph a 180-pound person burns 357 Calories per hour. Thus, in two hours a 180-pound person would burn 2 x 357 = 714 Calories.

But from this we must subtract the number of calories a 180-pound person would have used anyway if, instead of walking, he or she just sat for the two hours. From Table 5 this amounts to 105 Calories per hour, or 210 Calories in two hours. Then the net energy a 180-pound person would expend walking (over and above just sitting) totals 714 − 210 = 504 Calories.

However, the woman in this example weighs 187 pounds and would expend proportionately more calories than a 180-pound person, or 504 x 187/180 = **524 Calories**

## Types of Exercise

Simply stated there are **three basic types of exercise: aerobic, stretching, and strengthening**.

**Aerobic exercises** (also called "cardio") condition your cardiovascular system. Aerobic exercises, such as jogging, swimming, cycling, brisk walking, skipping rope, jogging in place, and many others, are typically deep breathing and continuous, with rhythmic and repetitive contractions of your large muscle groups. The main goal of an aerobic exercise

16

program is to increase the rate which your body can process oxygen, i.e., increase $VO_{2max}$. A well-conditioned person with efficient lungs and a strong heart can pump circulatory system effectively transport the oxygen in the air they breathe to all parts of their body.

| Activity | Weight (lbs.) | | | | | | | | |
|---|---|---|---|---|---|---|---|---|---|
| | 120 | 140 | 160 | 180 | 200 | 220 | 240 | 260 | 280 |
| Aerobics-dance | 491 | 573 | 655 | 736 | 818 | 900 | 982 | 1064 | 1145 |
| Basketball | 382 | 445 | 509 | 573 | 636 | 700 | 764 | 827 | 891 |
| Bicycle 13 mph | 435 | 508 | 580 | 653 | 725 | 798 | 870 | 943 | 1015 |
| Calisthenics | 341 | 398 | 455 | 511 | 568 | 625 | 682 | 739 | 795 |
| Dancing | 250 | 292 | 333 | 375 | 417 | 458 | 500 | 542 | 583 |
| Golf (pull cart) | 270 | 315 | 360 | 405 | 450 | 495 | 540 | 585 | 630 |
| Golf (riding) | 190 | 222 | 253 | 285 | 317 | 348 | 380 | 412 | 443 |
| Handball | 365 | 426 | 487 | 548 | 609 | 670 | 731 | 792 | 853 |
| Hiking | 320 | 373 | 427 | 480 | 533 | 587 | 640 | 693 | 747 |
| Jog -8 min mile | 680 | 793 | 907 | 1020 | 1133 | 1247 | 1360 | 1473 | 1587 |
| Mowing lawn | 299 | 349 | 399 | 449 | 499 | 549 | 599 | 649 | 699 |
| Raking leaves | 328 | 383 | 438 | 493 | 547 | 602 | 657 | 711 | 766 |
| Rowing | 380 | 443 | 507 | 570 | 633 | 697 | 760 | 823 | 887 |
| Sitting | 70 | 82 | 93 | 105 | 117 | 128 | 140 | 152 | 163 |
| Skating | 380 | 443 | 507 | 570 | 633 | 697 | 760 | 823 | 887 |
| Ski +country | 435 | 508 | 580 | 653 | 725 | 798 | 870 | 943 | 1015 |
| Ski downhill | 330 | 385 | 440 | 495 | 550 | 605 | 660 | 715 | 770 |
| Skipping rope | 457 | 533 | 609 | 686 | 762 | 838 | 914 | 990 | 1067 |
| Soccer | 410 | 479 | 547 | 615 | 684 | 752 | 820 | 889 | 957 |
| Softball | 270 | 315 | 360 | 405 | 450 | 495 | 540 | 585 | 630 |
| Spinning | 382 | 445 | 509 | 573 | 636 | 700 | 764 | 827 | 891 |
| Squash | 365 | 426 | 487 | 548 | 609 | 670 | 731 | 792 | 853 |
| Swimming laps | 440 | 513 | 587 | 660 | 733 | 807 | 880 | 953 | 1027 |
| Tennis-singles | 320 | 373 | 427 | 480 | 533 | 587 | 640 | 693 | 747 |

| Tennis-doubles | 243 | 283 | 324 | 364 | 405 | 445 | 485 | 526 | 566 |
|---|---|---|---|---|---|---|---|---|---|
| Walk 3 mph | 194 | 227 | 259 | 291 | 324 | 356 | 388 | 421 | 453 |
| Walk 3.5 mph | 238 | 277 | 317 | 357 | 396 | 436 | 476 | 515 | 555 |
| Walk 4 mph | 302 | 353 | 403 | 453 | 504 | 554 | 604 | 655 | 705 |

**Table 5: Calories Burned vs. Activity**

Regular aerobic exercise "trains" the heart to pump more blood with less effort. Aerobic exercise improves the circulatory system by developing more elastic arteries and by creating peripheral or extra blood paths to the heart; and aerobic exercise strengthens the muscles of respiration increasing the volume of oxygen that can be processed within a given time. Done regularly, aerobic exercises improve stamina and endurance, and most importantly promote what should be your central exercise goal - cardiovascular fitness. For if your cardiovascular system is not in shape, you're not in shape - no matter how many push-ups or crunches you can do!

**Stretching-type exercises** such as yoga, tai chi, Pilates and to a lesser extent calisthenics can improve your flexibility – and some of the exercises can make you somewhat stronger.

As you age you inevitably start to loose flexibility. Your gait becomes stiffer; you can't stand quite as upright as you used to; it becomes tougher to bend over; and you have difficulty turning your neck. Regardless of your age, however, stretching can make you more flexible, less injury prone, and can reduce the pain and discomfort associated with tight muscles and shortened tendons. Realize, however, that stretching exercises do not condition your heart and lungs. Stretching exercises are fine as long as they are performed in addition to rather than in place of an aerobic exercise.

Most experts do recommend stretching before and after aerobic and strength routines. However, never stretch cold muscles and always do some form of warm up prior to stretching. Stretch slowly and hold gently. You should stretch to the point of feeling a mild pull, but you should never feel pain. And when you stretch – do not bounce.

**Muscle building and strengthening exercises,** e.g., weight lifting, use of the machines found in fitness centers and isometrics.

Once more, as you age you loose muscle mass, your bone density decreases and you lose strength. Exercises like weight lifting strengthen your muscles, bones and joints. Strengthening exercises also reduce your

18

risk of developing osteoporosis, a severe bone-loss disease, which can lead to easily fractured bones and all the complications that often follow. Strong muscles not only allow you to lug groceries up to a second floor apartment, but as with increased flexibility, strong muscles also make you less injury prone. **Strengthening exercises are beneficial and should be a part of your fitness routine**, **but again they should be performed in addition to an aerobic exercise** because alone they cannot condition your heart and lungs.

## Select the Right Exercise

Selecting the right fitness exercise is the key to a successful conditioning program. You should pick an activity (or activities) you will enjoy. You may decide to concentrate on one activity such as squash, or you may choose to walk briskly some days and lift weights on other days. Incidentally, three to five days of a vigorous aerobic exercise plus two days of either strength or flexibility exercises per week is a good combination. Whatever you settle on make sure it is an activity that can be done regularly and that you enjoy. Factors to consider in choosing your activity are:

<u>Your Medical Condition</u>:  If you have a medical condition such as a heart problem, diabetes, osteoporosis, etcetera, or you should proceed with caution, and be sure to talk to your doctor before you start any exercise activity.

<u>Your Fitness Level</u>: If you have been inactive for some time, rather than starting with one of the more strenuous exercises, **beginners of all ages should initially confine themselves to walking** until they can easily walk two miles at a brisk pace. When you reach this stage more strenuous exercises can be attempted if desired. Furthermore, some sports medicine physicians contend that **if you are badly overweight you should limit your exercise to walking** until you have lost weight to the point where you are less than 25 percent overweight.

<u>Your Exercise Goals</u>:  If you want to strengthen your heart and lungs, improve your aerobic capacity and burn a lot of calories select an aerobic activity. If you want to improve your flexibility select a stretching type exercise. And if you want to become physically stronger choose one of the strength-building exercises.

<u>Your Schedule</u>: Only you know what the demands on your time from work, family and your social life are. What is the best time of day for you? Which days of the week best fit your schedule? Of course, you must

be open to rearranging your priorities to fit exercise into your daily life.

**Outdoors or Indoors:** If you decide to exercise outdoors you should also have an alternate indoor activity, an activity you can fall back on in bad weather. For example, if you choose to jog outside early in the morning before work, you may want to purchase a treadmill for use at home on days when it is either too hot, too cold or the weather is bad.

**Alone or with Others:** On the plus side, an exercise partner can make exercise more enjoyable and can help you get going and keep going on days when you might otherwise quit. On the other hand, a partner probably means that you have the schedules of two people to contend with and plan around, which can at times actually hinder your workout.

**How Much Are You Prepared to Spend:** For many activities, you will need little or no special equipment. For instance, walking outside only requires comfortable shoes; whereas, joining and working out at a fitness center can be relatively expensive.

## Aerobic Exercise: How Hard?

Because cardiovascular fitness should be your prime concern, **the central part of your exercise program should be an aerobic (or cardio) exercise done regularly**. Additional stretching and strengthening exercises should be included as time allows – but never to the exclusion of the aerobic portion of your program.

An aerobic exercise program should be vigorous enough to condition the cardiovascular system but not so strenuous as to exceed safe limits. I define safe as an exercise pace that is "comfortable." What they mean is that if, for instance, you are jogging or walking briskly you should be able to converse comfortably with a partner. You should be breathing and feeling normally within ten minutes after you stop exercising. If not you are exercising too vigorously. Other signs that you are pushing too hard include difficulty breathing, feeling faint, or feeling weak – during or after exercising. If you experience any of these symptoms, you are exercising too intensely and you should cut back.

Some experts prefer a more quantitative definition. They refer to the beneficial yet safe exercise region as the "Target Training Zone," or TTZ, which is determined by monitoring your pulse. The idea is to raise your pulse through exercise to a specific range (the target training zone) and hold it there for an extended period to obtain a cardiovascular benefit. On this concept rests the so-called heart-rated theory of exercise, which relies on heart rate (or pulse) to establish the proper exercise intensity.

## Aerobic Target-Training Zone

The **Target-Training Zone (TTZ) is a measure of aerobic exercise intensity**. Use the following procedure to calculate your TTZ:

**1)** Calculate your **Max heart rate** = 220 minus your Age. (Your maximum heart rate is the fastest your heart can beat, and you definitely must exercise well below this level.)

**2)** Compute your **Max heart rate reserve** = Max heart rate – Resting pulse.

**3)** Lastly, calculate your **TTZ** pulse = (Max heart rate reserve multiplied by Exercise intensity level) + Resting pulse.

If you would rather not do the mathematics, you may determine your TTZ from Tables 6 and 7 (on the following pages.) But before that, you need to determine the exercise intensity level that is right for you.

## Aerobic Exercise: Intensity-Level

Many exercise physiologists recommend the following guidelines:

**Low Exercise-Intensity Level**: This intensity level should be used by anyone over 50 years old, and by those starting a physical fitness program after many years of inactivity regardless of their age. People in this classification should begin exercising at 40 to 50% of their TTZ.

**Moderate Exercise-Intensity Level**: This applies to moderately active people who are under 50 years old and who, for example, have been walking two or three miles per day regularly. These men and women may begin exercising at 50 to 65% of their TTZ.

**High Exercise-Intensity Level**: This level applies to very active, well-trained, fit people under 50 years old. These individuals may exercise at 65 to 80% of their TTZ.

Keep in mind that these recommendations are aimed at the general population. In other words, they may not be right for you. Some people cannot raise their pulse, despite vigorous exercise, into their target-training zone. If you are one of these individuals, you probably have a maximum heart rate that is lower than average and so should disregard the target

| Age | Resting Pulse | Exercise Intensity (%) | | | | |
|---|---|---|---|---|---|---|
| | | 40 | 50 | 60 | 70 | 80 |
| 20 | 50 | 110 | 125 | 140 | 155 | 170 |
| | 60 | 116 | 130 | 144 | 158 | 172 |
| | 70 | 122 | 135 | 148 | 161 | 174 |
| | 80 | 128 | 140 | 140 | 164 | 176 |
| 25 | 50 | 108 | 123 | 137 | 152 | 166 |
| | 60 | 114 | 128 | 141 | 155 | 168 |
| | 70 | 120 | 133 | 145 | 158 | 170 |
| | 80 | 126 | 138 | 149 | 161 | 172 |
| 30 | 50 | 106 | 120 | 134 | 148 | 162 |
| | 60 | 112 | 125 | 138 | 151 | 164 |
| | 70 | 118 | 130 | 142 | 154 | 166 |
| | 80 | 124 | 135 | 146 | 157 | 168 |
| 35 | 50 | 104 | 118 | 131 | 145 | 158 |
| | 60 | 110 | 123 | 135 | 148 | 160 |
| | 70 | 116 | 128 | 139 | 151 | 162 |
| | 80 | 122 | 133 | 143 | 154 | 164 |
| 40 | 50 | 102 | 115 | 128 | 141 | 154 |
| | 60 | 108 | 120 | 132 | 144 | 156 |
| | 70 | 114 | 125 | 136 | 147 | 158 |
| | 80 | 120 | 130 | 140 | 150 | 160 |
| 45 | 50 | 100 | 113 | 125 | 138 | 150 |
| | 60 | 106 | 118 | 129 | 141 | 152 |
| | 70 | 112 | 123 | 133 | 144 | 154 |
| | 80 | 118 | 128 | 137 | 147 | 156 |

Table 6: TTZ: 20 to 45 year olds

| Age | Resting Pulse | Exercise Intensity (%) | | | | |
|---|---|---|---|---|---|---|
| | | 40 | 50 | 60 | 70 | 80 |
| 50 | 50 | 98 | 110 | 122 | 134 | 146 |
| | 60 | 104 | 115 | 126 | 137 | 148 |
| | 70 | 110 | 120 | 130 | 140 | 150 |
| | 80 | 116 | 125 | 134 | 143 | 152 |
| 55 | 50 | 96 | 108 | 119 | 131 | 142 |
| | 60 | 102 | 113 | 123 | 134 | 144 |
| | 70 | 108 | 118 | 127 | 137 | 146 |
| | 80 | 114 | 123 | 131 | 140 | 148 |
| 60 | 50 | 94 | 105 | 116 | 127 | 138 |
| | 60 | 100 | 110 | 120 | 130 | 140 |
| | 70 | 106 | 115 | 124 | 133 | 142 |
| | 80 | 112 | 120 | 128 | 136 | 144 |
| 65 | 50 | 92 | 103 | 113 | 124 | 134 |
| | 60 | 98 | 108 | 117 | 127 | 136 |
| | 70 | 104 | 113 | 121 | 130 | 138 |
| | 80 | 110 | 118 | 125 | 133 | 140 |
| 70 | 50 | 90 | 100 | 110 | 120 | 130 |
| | 60 | 96 | 105 | 114 | 123 | 132 |
| | 70 | 102 | 110 | 118 | 126 | 134 |
| | 80 | 108 | 115 | 122 | 129 | 136 |

**Table 7: TTZ: 50 to 70 year olds**

training zones shown here. Rather you should try to establish and be guided by a lower, more comfortable, exercising pulse range. If you do use the target-training zone approach, your pulse becomes your exercise guide. In addition, after a couple of months of aerobic exercise a sure indication that you are rounding into shape, making progress, is that your resting pulse slows down somewhat – especially if it was relatively fast at the start. This is because well-conditioned strengthened hearts are more efficient and so beat more slowly at rest. Trained athletes often have a resting pulse of 50 beats per minute or lower, whereas the "average" pulse is 72 to 76 for untrained men and 75 to 80 for untrained women. Furthermore, understand that as you become more physically fit you will have to exercise more vigorously to get your exercising pulse rate into your target-training zone.

**Example**:  Determine the target-training zone (TTZ) for a 40-year old relatively inactive woman with a resting pulse of 70, whose physician has approved her intention to start an aerobic exercise program.

Because she is relatively inactive but also relatively young, following the exercise-intensity level guidelines outlined earlier, she determines that she may start her exercise program at about 50 percent of her maximum heart rate reserve.  She determines her (TTZ) as follows:

**Max heart rate** = 220 - Age = 220 - 40 = 180
**Max heart rate reserve** = Max heart rate – Resting pulse = 180 – 70 = 110
**TTZ** = (Max heart rate reserve multiplied by Exercise intensity level) +
Resting pulse  = (110 x 0.50) + 70 = <u>125 beats per minute</u>
(Note, the exercise-intensity level converted from 50 % to the decimal equivalent 0.50.)

Alternatively, the 40-year old woman could have used Table 6, where first she would search the far left side of the table and locate her age (40).  Then from the four possible resting pulse selections she would choose (70); finally she would run her finger horizontally (to the right) until it intersects the vertical column headed by the 50 percent exercise intensity level where she would find her TTZ of 125 beats per minute. Because it is difficult to get an exact pulse during or immediately after exercising and this is not an exact science, she should convert her calculated TTZ into a TTZ range.  In this case, for a 50 percent exercise intensity level her TTZ range would be about 122 to 128 beats per minute.

## Aerobic Exercise:  How Often?

The American College of Sports Medicine recommends that an exercise heart rate of 60 to 90 percent of your maximum heart rate should be maintained for about 30 to 45 minutes three to five days per week to become reasonably fit.  They also stated, "For most people exercising at the lower end of their heart rate range for a longer time is better than exercising at the higher end of the range for a shorter time."  The United States Surgeon General recommends that people accumulate 30 minutes of moderate activity on most, if not all, days of the week.  More recently, the U.S. Institute of Medicine suggested 60 minutes of moderate exercise every day.  To confuse matters even more, many exercise physiologists favor the following exercise schedule:

**Low Exercise-Intensity Level** (40 to 50% of maximum heart rate reserve): People in this category (because of their age or lack of fitness) should work up to exercising 60 minutes per day at least five days per week. Despite the low intensity exercise level participants should achieve what exercise physiologists feel is an acceptable – albeit minimum – level of fitness.

**Moderate Exercise-Intensity Level** (50 to 65% of maximum heart rate reserve): Men and women at this level should build up to 45 minutes of exercise per day at least five days per week to achieve a minimum fitness level.

**High Exercise-Intensity Level** (65 to 80% of maximum heart rate reserve): In this category, individuals should work up to 30 minutes of exercise per day at least five days per week for a minimally acceptable fitness level.

As you can see, in general if you exercise at the lower exercise intensity levels your workout should last longer. Moreover, the longer and more frequently you exercise the greater your fitness reward. How fit you become is really a matter of your age, your genes, how fit you think you should be – and how hard you are willing to work. **But don't overdo it**! Again, it is worth repeating, everyone should have medical clearance before beginning any exercise program.

## Aerobic Exercise: Typical Workout

First, do not smoke before you exercise (or after for that matter); do not eat for two hours before you start exercising, and refrain from drinking any alcohol for four hours prior to beginning your exercise routine. **A classic aerobic exercise routine consists of a warm up, your main exercise, and a cool down.**

- Start with a three to seven minute warm up. Three minutes of stretching is sufficient if you are going to engage in a low intensity Group C exercise such as badminton; whereas a longer seven-minute warm up is better preparation for a high intensity Group A aerobic exercises such as jogging, cycling or stair climbing.

- Then move on to 30 to 60 minutes of your main aerobic exercise.

- Finish with a three to seven minute cool down period. Once more, if you are finishing a low-intensity exercise three minutes is enough. After a moderate or high-intensity aerobic exercise a seven minute cool down is more appropriate.

**Warm up:** Going from a resting state to a moderate or high-intensity exercise is a large jump. The warm up period gives your body time to bridge the gap and get ready for the more strenuous exercise that follows. Tension in your muscles and nerves is released; your large-frame muscles, ligaments and joints are stretched and put through their full range of motion; and your arteries and capillaries start to dilate as your heart beats faster and your blood-flow rate increases.

Begin your warm up by walking slowly and gradually increase your pace as you approach the end of the warm up period. Next stretch. **Never stretch cold muscles**. Many stretches are based on yoga, where you start with good posture and then use your body weight to stretch your tissues. The following is a list of stretching exercises are especially suited for warm up and cool down periods. Stretches (c) through (g) are illustrated in Figure 1. (Some of these stretches can be done toward the end of the walking segment of your warm-up.) Perform the stretches as described.

**a) Neck Swivel**: From a standing position, with your arms hanging loosely, rotate your head about your neck, five times clockwise, then five times counter clockwise.

**b) Shoulder Roll**: While standing, with your arms hanging loosely at your side rotate your shoulders first in a forward motion, then backwards. Repeat five times.

**c) Arm Pumping**: Again, from a standing position, raise your elbows to shoulder height. Pull your elbows and arms slowly rearward as you thrust your chest forward. Repeat five times.

**d) Side to side Stretch**: From a standing position, raise both hands over your head. Bend slowly from side to side. Repeat five times.

**e) Toe Touch**: Sit along a bench and place your right leg on the bench. Position your left leg on the floor. Lean forward and try to touch your right toe until feel a stretch behind your right knee and calf. Do not bounce. Hold for a count of ten. Repeat with left leg raised. (This stretch can also be done from a standing position by placing a leg on a chair.)

**f) Wall Push to Stretch Calves**: Stand about two feet from a wall. Then as you extend your arms forward lean into the wall. Keep both heels flat on the floor. Do not bounce. Hold this position for a count of ten.

**g) Quad Stretch**: Balance yourself by placing your left hand on wall. Bend your right leg and move your right heel toward your rear. Grab your right foot with your right hand. Pull gently. You should feel mild pressure in your right quad (front of your right thigh). Do not bounce. Hold for a ten count. Repeat for left leg.

Do not feel limited to the preceding stretching exercises. There are many, many other good stretches available (too many to discuss here) that you might prefer.

If your main activity is a low-intensity exercise, you can conclude your warm up after stretching out. If you are going on to a moderate or high-intensity aerobic exercise, after stretching start your main aerobic

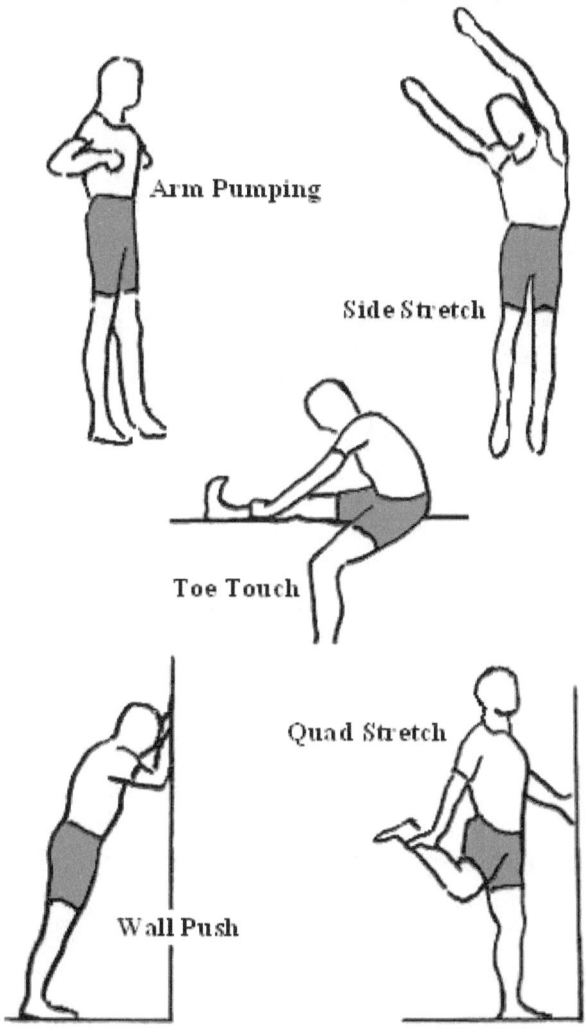

**Figure 1: Stretching Exercises**

exercise but at a relatively lower level. Over the next few minutes gradually increase the intensity so that your pulse approaches your target training zone. For instance, if you are a jogger you might warm up as follows: Start by walking slowly but steadily walk faster. After approximately five minutes stop and do two minutes of stretching. In theory, your warm up is over, but begin the main portion of your exercise by walking much faster, transition to a slow jog, then jog somewhat faster, and so on until, after about five minutes you have reached your regular jogging pace.

**Main Exercise:** Now you can begin your aerobic exercise of choice in earnest, stopping only to see that your pulse is in your target-training zone. If not, adjust your exercise level, exerting more or less effort. (Eventually, you will be able to sense that you are exercising at the correct intensity level and need only monitor your pulse occasionally.)

**Cool Down:** A five to seven-minute cooling off period should follow an aerobic workout. During cool down keep moving, decrease your activity level slowly. End your workout with leg stretches such as toe touches, a wall push and a quad stretch.

## Pulse Measurement

In order to monitor the intensity of exercise, you should occasionally stop during your workout and take your pulse immediately. This is because your pulse will fall quickly once you stop exercising. The trick is to find your pulse within a couple of seconds and then start counting.

Quickly place the tips of two fingers on one of the two carotid arteries in your neck. (Your carotid arteries are located on either side of your throat.) Count the beats for ten seconds and multiply by six. For example, if you count 20 beats in ten seconds then your pulse would be 120 beats per minute.

You are doing fine if your pulse is within your TTZ range. If your pulse is too slow, exercise somewhat harder; if your pulse is fast, exercise easier. Again, after you have exercised for some time you will be able to feel that you are exerting the correct amount of effort and need only check your exercising pulse about once a week. (Note: The best way to find your resting pulse is to measure it immediately upon rising in the morning. Use the average over three days for the truest result.)

## Walking Program

If your goal is to improve your general health and fitness, walking is a wonderful exercise. It's an exercise that you can do anywhere, that you can do outdoors or indoors, that requires no special equipment other than a good comfortable pair of walking shoes, and that you can do well into your old age. Walking does have a downside. Because it is a relatively low-intensity exercise, to get a good workout you have to spend more time walking compared to most high-intensity exercises.

If you are more than 50 years old, or have been sedentary for some time, it is best to start with a walking program that slowly but surely builds in intensity. If you walk hard enough, long enough and often enough, a walking workout can make you fit. Table 8, on the following page, shows a ten-week
beginner's walking routine.

The first session in week 1 starts cautiously with approximately three minutes of warm-up walking at a very easy pace of about 2.5 mph. Continue your warm up with two minutes of stretching. (See the stretching exercises described in Figure 1.) Then start walking more briskly, about 3.5 mph, but you should check your pulse and increase or decrease this to get your heart rate to a TTZ corresponding to about a 50 percent intensity level. After eight minutes, start your cool down by reducing your walking speed again to about 2.5 mph for three minutes. Conclude your session by doing about two minutes of stretching. The total workout time in week 1 is 18 minutes per session. The only part that changes in succeeding weeks (2 through 10), is the brisk walking portion of the workout increases continually from 8 minutes in week 1 to 30 minutes in week 10.

Walk at least three days a week for ten weeks. If you find a week particularly tiring, backup to the previous week (or repeat the week) before continuing with the program. This is not a contest; you do not have to finish the program in ten weeks. Once you complete the ten-week program you can either stay on a walking routine, or go on to one of the more strenuous aerobic exercises.

If you decide to become a walker and want to improve, first go from walking three days per week to five days per week – at the same TTZ. To improve further gradually increase your total workout time from 40 to 60 minutes. To improve even more, gradually increase your walking speed, and TTZ, so that your exercise intensity level approaches 60 percent. Another good way to increase the intensity of your walking workout is to include some hills in your route. Incidentally, as you would expect, walking over hilly terrain also burns more calories than walking on level ground.  On the two days you don't walk, try to get in 20 minutes of strengthening exercises.

| Week | Warm up (Minutes) | | Brisk Walking (Minutes) | Cool down (Minutes) | | Total Minutes |
|---|---|---|---|---|---|---|
| | Walk | Stretch | | Walk | Stretch | |
| 1 | 3 | 2 | 8 | 3 | 2 | 18 |
| 2 | 3 | 2 | 10 | 3 | 2 | 20 |
| 3 | 3 | 2 | 12 | 3 | 2 | 22 |
| 4 | 3 | 2 | 14 | 3 | 2 | 24 |
| 5 | 3 | 2 | 16 | 3 | 2 | 26 |
| 6 | 3 | 2 | 18 | 3 | 2 | 28 |
| 7 | 3 | 2 | 20 | 3 | 2 | 30 |
| 8 | 3 | 2 | 23 | 3 | 2 | 33 |
| 9 | 3 | 2 | 26 | 3 | 2 | 36 |
| 10 | 3 | 2 | 30 | 3 | 2 | 40 |

**Table 8: Walking Program for Beginners**

Because you will undoubtedly do most of your walking outside, you have to be aware of the weather forecast and have a backup plan for inclement weather.  On bad-weather days, you could use an indoor walking site (like a mall, or an indoor track), walk on a treadmill, or do stretching or strength exercises instead of walking.

## Get a Pedometer and Step Out

Sedentary people only take about 2,000 to 3,000 steps a day.  For the average person with a stride equal to about 2.5 feet (0.75 m), 2,100 steps amounts to walking about one mile (1.6 km). A Harvard University study has shown that 6,000 steps a day correlate with lower death rates in men, and that 8,000 to 10,000 step per day promote weight loss.  And these health and weight management benefits don't oblige you to walk continuously until you accrue the required number of steps.  Rather, all steps throughout the day to wherever and whenever count toward your daily total. (Some pedometers also show total "aerobic steps," correctly defined as those steps accumulated during at least 10 minutes of continuous walking at a rate of at least 60 steps per minute.)  Because 10,000 steps a day may not be achievable by some people, particularly by those who are elderly, sedentary, or who have chronic diseases, rather than insisting on a blanket 10,000 steps per day, a stepping goal should be based on an individual's baseline steps plus an increment of additional steps. (Your baseline is the number of steps taken in an average day.)

A pedometer keeps track of your steps. And a study by the American College of Sports Medicine found that participants who used pedometers were motivated to add about 2,000 steps to their daily routine. To start a stepping program, buy a pedometer. Wear the pedometer for a week and determine the number of steps you take on an average day. This is your baseline. Then add the equivalent of half an hour of walking to your day, or roughly 2,500 extra steps per day. For example, consider a woman who wears a pedometer and notes that on an average day she accumulates 3,500 steps. Her goal should be to add the equivalent of a half hour of walking to her day, or roughly 2,500 more steps per day, for a daily total of 6,000 steps.

There are many little ways to add steps to your day, such as taking stairs rather than an elevator, parking further from your destination, pacing as you talk on the telephone, marching-in-place for a minute once every hour – and of course taking short walks whenever you can. So buy a pedometer or get a pedometer app for your smart phone. Get off the couch and step out for your health!

**Pedometer Calibration:** Because pedometers count steps, to display the distance walked, you have to measure and then input your average step length. To do this walk a known distance with your pedometer in place and then divide the known distance by the number of steps. Generally, the longer the distance the more accurate the calibration. A local high school football field is a good calibration site, with a known 100 yards (300 feet) from goal line to goal line. In this case, to determine your average step length, divide 300 feet by the number of steps. Let's assume your pedometer indicated it took you 113 steps to cover the 300 feet. Then your average step length is 300 feet divided by 113 steps which equals 2.65 feet. (To enter this in most pedometers, you will have to convert this to 2' 8".)

## Jogging Program

If you are in reasonably good condition, have completed the "Walking Program for Beginners," or have been walking regularly, and have medical clearance, you can start a jogging program. Table 9, on the following page, illustrates a 13-week beginner's schedule. Try to get your pulse into your TTZ but don't overdue it. Gradually, over time, you want

31

to increase both the intensity and distance of your jogging routine. However, if you don't have the physical makeup to do both, always choose endurance over intensity; i.e., choose distance rather than speed, choose to jog longer rather than faster.

| Week | Warm up (Minutes) | | Brisk Walking & Jogging (Minutes) | Cool down (Minutes) | | Total Minutes |
|------|------|---------|------|------|---------|------|
| | Walk | Stretch | | Walk | Stretch | |
| 1 | 5 | 2 | Walk 5  Jog 3<br>Walk 5  Jog 3 | 3 | 2 | 28 |
| 2 | 5 | 2 | Walk 4  Jog 5<br>Walk 4  Jog 5 | 3 | 2 | 30 |
| 3 | 5 | 2 | Walk 4  Jog 5<br>Walk 4  Jog 5 | 3 | 2 | 30 |
| 4 | 5 | 2 | Walk 4  Jog 6<br>Walk 4  Jog 6 | 3 | 2 | 32 |
| 5 | 5 | 2 | Walk 4  Jog 7<br>Walk 4  Jog 7 | 3 | 2 | 34 |
| 6 | 5 | 2 | Walk 4  Jog 8<br>Walk 4  Jog 8 | 3 | 2 | 36 |
| 7 | 5 | 2 | Walk 4  Jog 9<br>Walk 4  Jog 9 | 3 | 2 | 38 |
| 8 | 5 | 2 | Walk 4  Jog 12 | 3 | 2 | 28 |
| 9 | 5 | 2 | Walk 4  Jog 15 | 3 | 2 | 31 |
| 10 | 5 | 2 | Walk 4  Jog 17 | 3 | 2 | 33 |
| 11 | 5 | 2 | Walk 2  Slow Jog 2<br>then Jog 17 | 3 | 2 | 33 |
| 12 | 5 | 2 | Walk 2  Slow Jog 4<br>then Jog 17 | 3 | 2 | 35 |
| 13 | 5 | 2 | Slow Jog 6<br>then Jog 17 | 3 | 2 | 35 |

**Table 9:  Jogging Program**

The first session in week 1 starts with approximately five minutes of walking at an easy pace of about 2.5 mph.  Continue your warm up with two minutes of stretching.  Then start walking more briskly, about 3.5

mph, but check your pulse and increase or decrease this to get your heart rate close to a TTZ that is roughly consistent with a 45 percent intensity level. After five minutes of brisk walking, jog for three minutes at a slightly higher heart rate, corresponding to about a 55 percent intensity level. Follow this with another five minutes of brisk walking and a three-minute jog. Cool down by walking again but now at an easy speed of about 2.5 mph for three minutes. Conclude your session by doing about two minutes of stretching. The total workout
time in week 1 is 26 minutes per session. In weeks 2 through 13, the time allotted to brisk walking decreases as the jogging time gradually increases.

Jog at least three days a week for 13 weeks. Again, if you find a week particularly tiring, backup to the previous week (or repeat the week) before continuing with the program. Once you complete the program, if you want to improve, first go from jogging three days per week to five days per week – at the same TTZ. To improve further gradually increase your total workout time from 30 to 60 minutes. To improve even more, gradually increase your jogging speed, and TTZ, so that your exercise intensity level approaches 65 percent. Another good way to increase the intensity of your jogging workout is to try to include some hills in your workout. On the two days you don't walk, try to get in 20 minutes of strengthening exercises.

Because you will undoubtedly do most of your jogging outside, you have to be aware of the weather forecast and have a contingency plan for inclement weather. On bad-weather days, you might use an indoor track, try an alternate exercise like jogging on a treadmill, or do stretching or strength exercises.

As always, stop exercising immediately if you experience tightness or pain in your chest, become lightheaded or dizzy, are severely breathless, lose muscle control or are nauseous. These are warning signs of over-exertion and you definitely should lower your exercise-intensity level. If you experience these symptoms, it is also a good idea to seek medical attention.

Be aware that the pounding your body gets from jogging usually takes its toll over time. Many joggers have recurring, nagging injuries, particularly to their legs and feet. If you begin to suffer chronic injuries,

remember there are other high-intensity aerobic exercises for which your body might be better suited. At that point, you might consider switching to cycling, a rowing machine, etc.

# Weight Lifting Speeds Your Metabolism

Strength-building exercises can increase your muscle mass, which tends to increase your basal metabolic rate – and helps you control your weight.

Of all the many strength-building options, I personally prefer free weights (actually dumbbells) because they can be used at home. Working out at home has some significant advantages. First, your workout takes less time because you don't have to drive back and forth to a fitness facility; second, you have the flexibility of dividing your workout into small time segments to fit your day, whenever you have time, such as when the baby is napping, and of course working out at home is certainly less expensive.

You can workout in a bedroom, basement, garage, attic – anywhere you have extra space. A set of variable (adjustable) weight dumbbells and a small weight bench don't take up much room and are all you need for a home-based gym. (Bear in mind, **knowledge and the discipline to work out regularly are far more important than fancy equipment**.) Before investing in a set of weights and a bench, however, it may still be worthwhile to start by joining a health club. At a health club you can get expert instruction on the use of free weights. And you may find that you actually prefer to workout at a club.

But if you do decide to opt for the convenience of a home-based gym, that would be the time to purchase a pair of variable-weight dumbbells and a strong weight bench (that will not tip over) for home use. Rather than an entire set of weights, purchase just enough dumbbell weight so that you can do a military press five times.

The seven dumbbell exercises that follow on pages 36 and 37 comprise a total-body workout, suitable for beginners, that involve all the major muscle groups. When done consecutively without stopping a series of exercises is called a circuit. To start, use the same dumbbell weight for all the exercises, a weight that allows you to do 10 to 15 repetitions of the most difficult exercise in the circuit. For the first week do one circuit per training session.

Your goal should be two circuits per session, which should take you about 20 minutes (with a two to three-minute rest between circuits). When you are comfortable at this level you are ready to increase the dumbbell weight – but by no more than roughly 10 percent (or one pound minimum). The seven exercises are illustrated in Figures 2 and 3. Perform 10 to 15 repetitions of each exercise.

**a) Bench Press**: With your head and back on the bench, hold a dumbbell in each hand to the side of your shoulders, palms facing each other. Slowly raise the dumbbells extending your arms above your shoulders. Pause, then lower the dumbbells down to the starting position. The bench press primarily works your pectorals, triceps and deltoids.

**b) One–Arm Dumbbell Row**: Hold a dumbbell in your right hand, palm facing toward your right thigh. Stand to the right of your weight bench and place your left knee on the bench. Support yourself by putting your left hand on the bench. (Flex your right knee slightly and lean forward so your back is almost parallel to the floor.) Slowly pull your right arm up until your upper arm is parallel to the floor. (Keep your right arm close to your torso.) Pause and lower your right arm to the starting position. After you complete a set, stand to the left of the bench and repeat the exercise with the dumbbell in your left hand. Rows mainly work your latissimus dorsi and rhomboid muscles.

**c) Seated Shoulder Press**: From a seated position, hold a dumbbell in each hand to the side of your shoulders, palms facing forward. Slowly raise the weights over your head until your arms are straight. Pause, then lower the dumbbells to the starting position. The shoulder press mainly exercises your deltoids, trapezius, triceps, latissimus dorsi and rhomboid muscles.

**d) Curls for Biceps**: Stand with a dumbbell in each hand, your arms hanging loosely, with your palms to the side your thighs and facing straight ahead. Keep your elbows tucked into your side and slowly lift the dumbbells until they are approximately shoulder high. Pause and lower the dumbbells to the starting position. Curls chiefly work your biceps.

**e) Tricep Extension**: With a dumbbell in your right hand, assume the same initial position as in the one-arm dumbbell row. Slowly move your right arm rearward until it is nearly parallel to the floor. Pause and then return the dumbbell to the starting position without bending your arm. After completing a set, stand to the left of the bench and repeat the exercise with the dumbbell in your left hand. This exercise mainly works your triceps.

**f) Front Squats**: Stand with a dumbbell in each hand, to the side of your shoulders, palms facing each other (inward). Slowly bend your knees to

**g) Curls for Abs**: This is not a weight lifting exercise but is a useful part of any routine. Lie face up on a floor mat with your hands folded over your chest and your legs bent. Keeping your feet flat on the mat, slowly curl your torso up and toward your thighs until your shoulder blades are

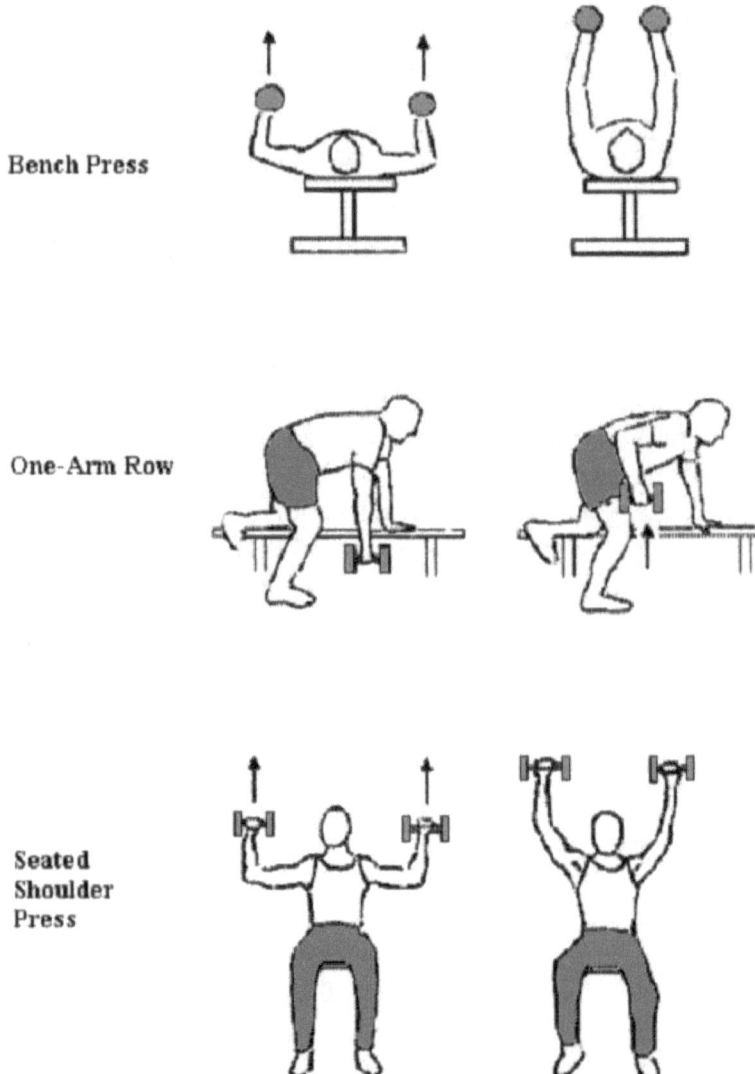

**Bench Press**

**One-Arm Row**

**Seated Shoulder Press**

**Figure 2:  Strengthening Exercises (a to c)**

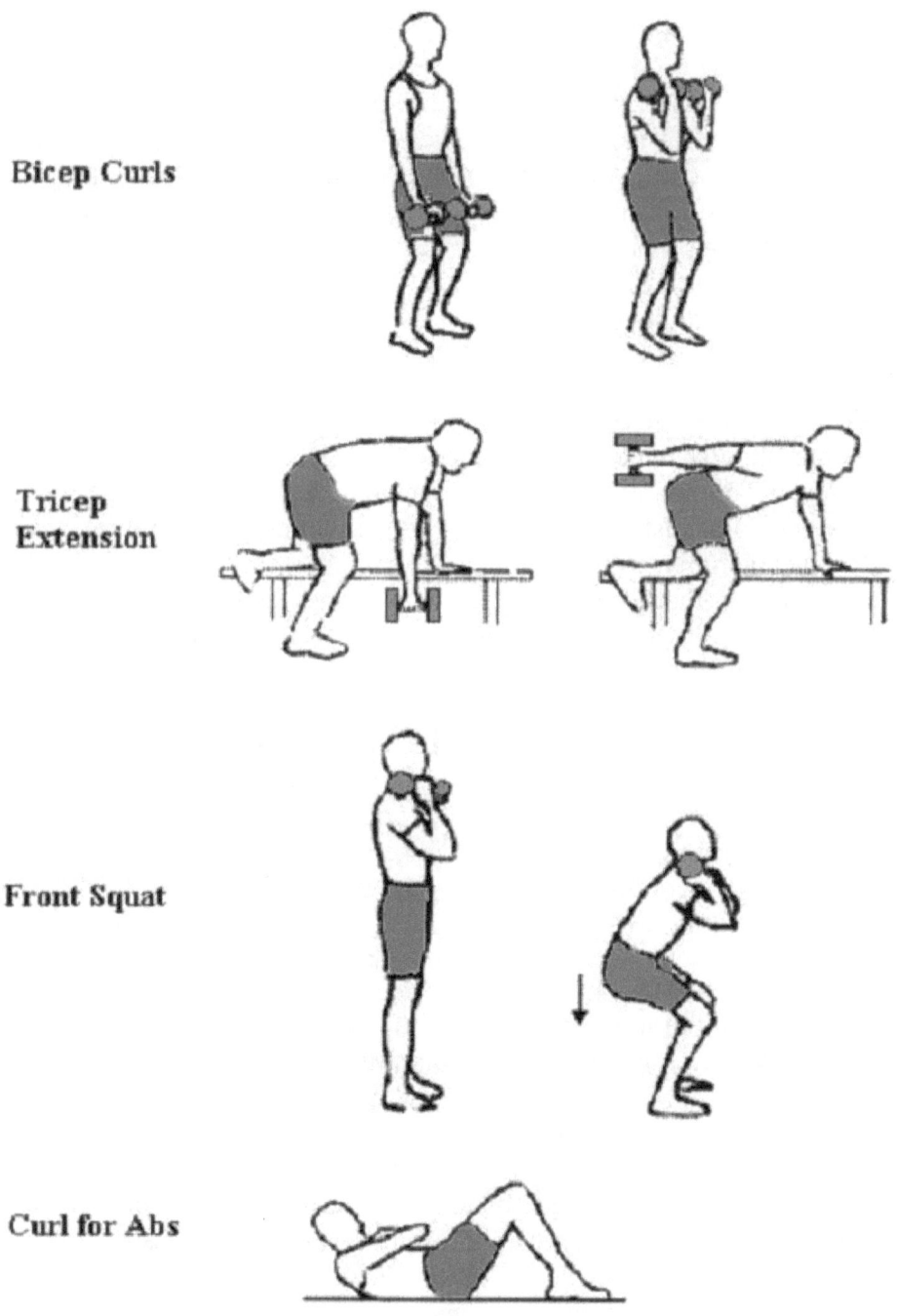

**Bicep Curls**

**Tricep Extension**

**Front Squat**

**Curl for Abs**

**Figure 3: Strengthening Exercises (d to g)**

off the mat. Pause, then return to the starting position. This exercise works your rectus abdominis muscles – your abs.

Remember to do about five minutes of aerobic and stretching exercises before and after your strength exercises, and to workout two to three (non-consecutive) days per week. Why non-consecutive days? Because strengthening exercises work a muscle until it's fatigued, and a day off is needed for muscles to recover, repair and rebuild. And listen to your body to determine your level of exertion. Don't over do it!

A final word about breathing properly: Never hold your breath during weight training. This can cause your blood pressure to get dangerously high. Rather, breathe naturally and try to exhale during a lift.

## Other Exercises

There are literally hundreds of other aerobic, flexibility and strengthening exercises. Too many to review here, but many are definitely worth considering. For instance, swimming laps in a pool provides an excellent low-impact aerobic workout that also builds strength. Of course, the disadvantage is that you need to join a fitness facility that has a pool. Some trainers think a good rowing machine, such as the Concept II, provides a great total-body workout. Others feel a workout on a stairclimber is hard to beat. All have advantages and disadvantages.

In fact, most trainers recommend that you modify your routine every few months to add variety. Some advocate alternating exercises every other session. For instance, if you jog and lift weights on alternate days, you avoid repeating movements on consecutive days. As bonus, you will also most likely avoid the injuries that are often associated with day-after-day repetitive motion.

## Missed Workouts

Inevitably, you will miss some aerobic or strengthening workouts. It may be because you're traveling, or due to a minor illness, or an injury. If you are ill or injured, wait for the injury to heal, or until you feel like your normal self before resuming your exercise routine. If you only miss a day or two, you can undoubtedly just pick up where you left off as if nothing happened. If you miss a week or more, however, you will probably have lost some of your fitness gains and might have to resume at a somewhat lower exercising-intensity level. This means that when you come back after missing some aerobic sessions, you might have to exercise at a slightly lower TTZ, or shorten the duration of your workout. And when you return after missing some strengthening sessions, you might want to reduce the weight you are lifting or reduce the number of repetitions.

Incidentally, physical fitness can be maintained only by regular workouts. If your exercise frequency drops to one day a week, half your fitness gains will be lost in 10 weeks. If exercise is stopped completely, virtually all your accumulated fitness benefits will be lost in five weeks! Therefore, if you want to keep that state of well-being, feeling better, looking better, it's important to make regular exercise part of your lifestyle.

## Exercise Risks and Problems

Certain situations may occur that indicate you may be doing too much, exercising too hard. A feeling of having worked hard is fine, sweating is good, but not a feeling of undo fatigue.

Perhaps the most frequent problems faced by exercisers are injuries of the joints and muscles: sprains and strains, knee pain, elbow pain, back pain, neck pain, shin splints and stress fractures. Most happen when you exercise too hard.

Potentially serious problems are signaled if you experience any of the following symptoms during or after exercise. The symptoms include but are not limited to any abnormal heart action such as an irregular heart rhythm; pain or pressure in the middle of your chest; pain in an arm or your neck; dizziness, fainting or lightheadedness; severe exhaustion; sudden loss of coordination; or confusion. If any of these symptoms are experienced, stop exercising immediately and get medical help.

## Avoiding Injury

When he practiced, my friend and workout buddy Dr. Kanaar's specialty was rehabilitation medicine but he also preached what he called "preventive medicine," that is avoiding injury by practicing a common-sense approach to exercise:

1) Have a medical checkup and set realistic fitness goals.
2) Build up your exercise intensity gradually over many weeks, months.
3) After you eat a meal, wait two hours before exercising.
4) Buy good suitable clothing for your exercise routine.
5) Use safety and protective equipment when appropriate, such as helmet when you bicycle, and goggles when you play handball, squash or racquetball.
6) Don't exercise outside on very hot day or very cold days.

**7)** If you insist on working out in very hot or cold weather, always let someone know when and where you will be exercising and when you are planning to return.

**8)** If you insist on working out in very hot or cold weather, always let someone know when and where you will be exercising and when you are planning to return.

**9)** If you are new to a gym or health club, attend an orientation session before you use any unfamiliar exercise equipment. Otherwise, read the operating instructions and ask someone qualified to help you.

**10)** For aerobic activities, warm up slowly to reach your TTZ and cool down slowly after you exercise.

**11)** Do not increase the difficulty of any activity (e.g., your walking or jogging distance, the amount of weight you lift) by more than 10 percent per week.

**12)** Jog on softer surfaces such as a level grass field, a dirt path, or a running track.

**13)** After exercising wait 30 minutes before eating.

**14)** As a final point, if you experience some early warning pain stop exercising.

**Minor Leg Injures**: Many minor leg injuries can be treated using the well-known **R.I.C.E**. method, i.e., rest, ice, compression, elevation.

- **Rest.** You may not have to avoid all physical activity; just take it easy.
- **Ice.** Apply ice for 15 minutes several times a day when there is swelling.
- **Compress** the area with a bandage or sleeve to help control swelling.
- **Elevate** the injured area above the level of your heart.

## My Exercise Routine

I started jogging in the late 1960's. Of course I was much younger then. I jogged three to five miles almost every morning and worked out with free weights (dumbbells) on the days I didn't jog. After 20 years of jogging, the constant pounding resulted in a troubling number of chronic minor leg and foot injuries. So I switched to walking and I have been walking ever since. Now I'm a semi-retired senior citizen. I have more time. For the past 15 years, from 6:00 to 7:00 am, I take a brisk walk covering slightly less than four miles. Most days I walk outside but when the weather is bad I head for a nearby shopping mall. For variety, some days I power walk in place for about 45 minutes using an exercise DVDs to set a rhythm; then I complete my workout doing two circuits of the dumbbell exercises described earlier.

In warmer weather I golf (walking 9 or 18 holes) or hike (about eight miles) two or three times a week. When I'm not golfing or hiking I go on my early morning walk. When I golf or hike – that's my workout. Although recently after I finished my brisk one-hour morning walk followed by 20 minutes of dumbbell exercises, a friend called later in the day and next thing I know I'm playing 18 holes of golf – walking of course. In total, I exercised 5 hours and 45 minutes, burned about 2000 Calories, and felt strong, definitely not tired, at the end of the day. Not bad for a 75 year-old senior!

In summary, one day I walk outside for an hour; the following day I power walk in place for 40 minutes using an exercise DVD and also lift weights; the next day I'm back to walking outside again; and so on. I've been doing this for 15 years. I exercise every day without fail. Every day! My exercise routine combined with a sensible diet have kept me trim over the years, within three pounds of my college-graduation weight. Most people think I'm much younger than my chronological age – and I feel great!

# NUTRITION FUNDAMENTALS

Nutrition is a crucial element of weight maintenance. Healthy eating habits, the result of sensible nutritional practices, must be an integral part of your weight maintenance program. In this section you will learn how to improve the "nutritional quality" of the food you eat, and foods you should avoid, i.e., those foods that are loaded with "nutritionally-empty calories."

## Are You Eating Properly?

To broadly assess how appropriate your current nutritional practices are please complete the following questionnaire. Then add up your point total.

**a) Number of vegetable servings eaten per day?** None (1 point), 1 serving (2 points), 2 to 4 (3 points), 5 or more (4 points)

**b) How many fruit servings do you eat in a day?** None (1 point), 1 serving (2 points), 2 to 4 (3 points), 5 or more (4 points)

**c) Cereal & whole-grain bread servings in a day?** None (1 pt), 1 serving (2 pts), 2 to 4 (3 pts), 5 or more (4 pts)

**d) How many times per week do you eat a fish or poultry?** Never (1 pt), 1 time (2 pts), 2 to 3 (3 pts), 4 or more (4 pts)

**e) How do you prepare and eat poultry?** Fry dark meat with skin & gravy (1 pt), Bake or broil dark meat with skin & gravy (2 pts), Bake or broil dark meat without skin (3 pts), Bake or broil white meat without skin (4 pts)

**f) How many times per week do you eat beans, lentils, peas?** Never (1 pt), 1 time (2 pts), 2 to 3 (3 pts), 4 or more (4 pts)

**g) How often per week do you eat hamburger, salami, frankfurter, bacon, etc?** 7 or more (1 pt), 4 to 6 (2 pts), 2 to 3 (3 pts), Rarely (4 pts)

**h) When you consume milk, yogurt, ice cream, etc, you most often select:** Only whole-fat dairy product (1 pt), Whole milk, but low-fat yogurt and ice cream (2 pts), Low-fat (1 or 2% fat) (3 pts), Skim or non-fat products (4 pts)

**i) If ordering potatoes in a restaurant you choose:** French fried or hash brown (1 pt), Baked or boiled with butter and/or sour cream (2 pts), Boiled w/o butter or sour cream (3 pts), Baked w/o butter or sour cream (4 pts)

**j) How many times per week do you eat fast-food?** 5 or more (1 pt), 3 or 4 times (2 pts), 1 or 2 (3 pts), Rarely (4 pts)

**k) Do you add salt to your food?** At every meal (1 pt), Once per day (2 pts), 2 or 3 times per week (3 pts), Rarely (4 pts)

**l) Do you eat sweets (cookies, candy bar, etc)?** More than one sweet per day (1 pt), About one per day (2 pts), 2 to 4 sweets per week (3 pts), Rarely (4 pts)

**m) Do you take any vitamin or mineral supplements?** None (1 pt), Take herbal supplements (2 pts), Take individual vitamins (like C, E, etc) (3 pts), Take multi-vitamin and mineral supplement (4 pts)

**n) If you want to lose weight, how do you proceed?** Go on a crash die (1 pt), Stop eating carbs (2 pts), Cut back on carbs & increase exercise (3 pts), Reduce caloric intake & increase exercise (4 pts)

This completes our brief nutrition practices assessment. Add up your score and see how you compare to the following standards.

- **49 to 56 points**. Excellent! You can definitely skip the following Nutrition sections and go directly to "**Become a Calorie Expert,**" on page 68.
- **41 to 48 points** Good. You can probably skip most of the following Nutrition sections and go to page 68.
- **32 to 40 points** Fair. You should read the Nutrition sections before proceeding.
- **14 to 31 points** Poor. You must read the Nutrition sections before proceeding.

## Healthy Eating

Healthy eating habits, the result of sensible nutritional practices, must be an integral part of your weight maintenance program. In this section you will learn how to improve the "nutritional quality" of the food you eat, and, as expected, we will also point out foods that you should avoid, i.e., those foods that are loaded with "nutritionally-empty calories."

Food is far more than just an energy source. Foods are made up of seven basic constituents: carbohydrates, proteins, fats, vitamins, minerals, fiber and water. For a healthy body you need to eat the correct quantity and proportion of all these components. You need protein, carbohydrates and fats, for growth, repair and energy. You need vitamins and minerals, albeit in relatively small quantities, so they can perform their vital roles in the thousands of biochemical reactions in your body. Fiber, the broad name given to the stuff you eat that your body cannot digest, is needed to assist your digestive system.

Fortunately, supermarkets have all the foods we need – and in abundance. Yet most nutritionists agree that a great many Americans are not eating well enough to sustain good health. In general, our diet is too high in fat – with an average of 40 percent of our calories from fat – contributing to atherosclerosis. Another culprit is sugar. As a nation we consume more than 100 pounds of sugar per year per person, totaling an unhealthy, nutritionally empty, 500 Calories per day. This large intake of sugar leads to obvious ills, such as obesity and tooth decay.

Add to this the increased use of processed and convenience foods, the proliferation of nutritional misinformation and deceptive advertising, and it is clear that most people must improve their understanding of nutrition in order to eat properly.

## Proteins are Building Blocks

Proteins are molecules of amino acids that are required for cell maintenance and repair, as well as for the regulation of a wide range of bodily functions. Humans need 22 amino acids in order to live. Our bodies can make 14 of the amino acids on their own, but eight of them, named the essential-amino acids, must be acquired from the foods we eat.

Some foods have all the amino acids needed to build other proteins. These are called complete proteins. Nearly every animal food, including dairy products, eggs, meat, poultry and fish are complete proteins because they contain all eight-essential amino acids. **Soy is the only plant-based food that has all eight essential-amino acids.**

Other plant-based protein sources lack one or more essential amino acids (i.e., amino acids that the body can neither create nor manufacture by modifying other amino acids.) These incomplete proteins are found in legumes, grains, nuts, and seeds. However, consuming combinations of foods that have incomplete proteins can provide the same complete protein end effect as animal protein. For a complete-protein meal, simply eat any of the incomplete plant proteins with another but different incomplete plant protein. Examples of some healthy plant-protein combinations that result in complete proteins are:

**Eat grains with legumes:** pasta & beans, rice & lentils, tortillas with refried beans, etc

**Eat grains with nuts or seeds:** such as peanut butter on whole-grain bread, etc

Around the world, millions of people do not get enough protein. Protein malnutrition can cause growth failure, loss of muscle mass, decreased immunity, weakening of the heart and respiratory system, and in some cases death. Whereas, in the United States and other developed countries, getting the minimum daily requirement of protein is usually not a problem, because almost any reasonable diet will provide most of us with sufficient protein.

Adults need about 0.79 grams of protein for every kilogram of body weight per day to keep from slowly breaking down their own tissue. (That translates to approximately 0.36 grams of protein for every pound of body weight.) A case in point, an adult weighing 154 pounds (70 kg) requires about (154 x 0.36), or 55 grams of protein per day. How much protein is in food? A few examples: There are approximately seven grams of protein per ounce of beef, poultry, fish, cheese or peanuts. Soybeans pack 10 grams of protein per ounce. Most other beans and lentils contain about six grams of protein per ounce. There are roughly three grams of protein in an ounce of whole-grain cereal, and milk has one gram of protein per fluid ounce.

Understand that foods are rarely straight protein. Some high-protein foods, such as marbled beef and whole milk, also come with lots of unhealthy saturated fat. Therefore, when you eat meat, eat the leanest cuts, and when you consume dairy products, choose skim or low-fat varieties. On the other hand, beans, nuts, and whole grains offer high-quality (albeit incomplete) protein with little saturated fat – but with lots of healthful fiber and micronutrients.

## You Need Carbs

Carbohydrates provide your body with its basic fuel, the energy your cells need to survive. The staple of most diets around the world, carbohydrates provide essential vitamins and minerals, fiber, and numerous beneficial compounds (phytonutrients) that promote good health.

The simplest carbohydrate is glucose. Glucose, also called "blood sugar" and "dextrose," flows in the bloodstream so that it is available to every cell in your body. Your body's cells absorb glucose and convert it into energy to drive the cell. Glucose is a simple sugar, meaning that it tastes sweet. Some other simple sugars are sucrose, also known as "white sugar," fructose, the main sugar in fruits, and lactose, the sugar found in milk. They all taste sweet, and most are digested and enter your bloodstream quickly. When you eat fruit or drink milk, however, the natural sugar comes with vitamins, minerals (and fiber in the case of fruit); whereas the simple sugars in candy, for instance, are nothing but nutritionally-empty calories.

Then there are the more complex carbohydrates. Most grains (wheat, corn, oats, rice) and foods like potatoes, pasta and plantains are complex carbohydrates. In general, but not always, complex carbohydrates are digested more slowly than simple carbohydrates, and take much longer to enter your bloodstream. Most of us have heard that eating complex carbohydrates is good, and eating sugar-loaded foods is a bad. The reason is that simple sugars require little digestion, and when you eat a sweet food, such as a candy bar, or drink a can of soda, your blood glucose level rises rapidly. In response, your pancreas secretes a large amount of insulin to keep your blood glucose levels from rising too high. The large insulin response in turn tends to cause your blood sugar to fall to levels that are too low. As a consequence, about three to five hours after consuming sweets you feel lethargic and hungry. Many people react to this by eating yet another sweet, which can start a rollercoaster ride of surging glucose and then insulin. None of this is experienced after eating most complex carbohydrates, or a balanced meal, because the digestion and absorption processes are much slower.

In summary, **carbohydrates are neither all good nor all bad.** Remember good carbohydrates provide needed micronutrients. You should try to get the bulk of your calories from the good carbohydrates, i.e., from fruits, from vegetables and from whole grains such as whole-grain cereal, whole-wheat bread, whole-grain pasta, whole-old-fashioned oats, brown rice, bulgur, millet, and hulled barley.

## Fats in Foods

Fats are found in vegetable oil, seeds and nuts, meat and fish, and dairy products, as well as in foods like potato chips and French fries (that are cooked in oil), cookies, cake, and so on. There are certain fats you absolutely need to survive (the essential-fatty acids), and others you would do well to drastically limit (saturated fats) or avoid altogether (trans fats). Chemically, all fatty acids contain carbon chains with hydrogen atoms bonded to the carbon, and all fats have the highest calorie density – containing nine calories per gram (more on this later).

Until recently, the best wisdom was to eat a low-fat, low-cholesterol diet. This advice is now largely out of date. The latest research seems to show that the total amount of fat in the diet may not be linked with disease. **What really matters is the type of fat in your diet.**

<u>Saturated Fats</u>: When all carbon bonds of a fat molecule are filled with hydrogen, a fat is said to be saturated, i.e., saturated with hydrogen atoms. Most saturated fats are animal in origin and are solid at room temperature (good examples are butter and the fat in meats). Generally speaking, you should avoid or at least severely limit your intake of saturated fats because they can raise both your total and bad LDL blood cholesterol levels which increases your chances of getting heart disease.

When hydrogen atoms are missing along the carbon chain the fatty acids are called monounsaturated or polyunsaturated depending on their exact chemical structure.

<u>Monounsaturated fats</u> (also called omega-9 fatty acids) are liquid at room temperature and are known as oils. They are "good fats" and are derived from plant sources, such as vegetable oils, nuts, and seeds. In studies in which monounsaturated fats were eaten in place of carbohydrates, LDL blood cholesterol levels decreased and HDL cholesterol levels increased. Monounsaturated fats are found in high concentrations in canola, olive and peanut oils.

<u>Polyunsaturated fats</u> are also liquid oils at room temperature and in your refrigerator. They are "good fats" and are derived from plant sources, such as vegetable oils, nuts, and seeds. Again, research has demonstrated that when polyunsaturated fats were eaten in place of carbohydrates, LDL blood cholesterol levels decreased and HDL cholesterol levels increased. Polyunsaturated fats are found in high concentrations in sunflower, soybean and corn oils.

<u>Essential-Fatty Acids</u> are class of polyunsaturated fatty acids that our body cannot create. These fats must be obtained from the food you eat. Essential-fatty acids promote absorption of the fat-soluble vitamins A, D, E, and K and are also thought to provide many disease-fighting benefits. Because essential-fatty acids are needed and our body cannot manufacture them, they must come from the food we eat. Essential-fatty acids fall into two groups: omega-3 and omega-6.

<u>Omega-3 fatty acids</u> are relatively hard to find. Foods high in omega-3 fatty acids are walnuts, tofu, flax seeds and oily fish (salmon, mackerel, sardines, trout and albacore tuna). Omega-3 fats are thought to be heart-protective. (The American Heart Association suggests that people with coronary-heart disease consult with their physician regarding

the advisability of taking a fish-oil supplement.)

**Omega-6 fatty acids**, on the other hand, are more common, easier to find, and are in most oils including sunflower, soybean and corn oils.

Current thinking is that the consumption of omega-6 and omega-3 fatty acids should be in the ratio of 3:1, with about three omega-6 for one omega-3. Many Western diets, however, contain about 15:1, omega-6 to omega-3, which is not good for your health. Although you need omega-6, people generally eat too much of it and not enough omega-3 fat. The American Heart Association recommends that you eat fish (particularly fatty fish) two times a week, as a way to get a more appropriate quantity of omega-3 fatty acids in your diet.

| Fat Type | Where found |
|---|---|
| Saturated | Meat, poultry (especially the skin), dairy products, lard, coconut oil, palm oil, cocoa butter |
| Trans Fats | Fried foods, margarine, snack foods, commercially-baked cake and cookies, and fast foods |
| Cholesterol | Egg yokes, dairy products, organ meats, fatty and prime meats, poultry skin, shellfish, shrimp |
| Polyunsaturated (Omega-3) | Mackerel, salmon, sardines, tuna, canola oil, walnuts, flaxseed, wheat germ |
| Polyunsaturated (Omega-6) | Corn oil, cottonseed oil, safflower oil, sunflower oil, soybean oil |
| Monounsaturated (Omega-9) | Canola oil, olive oil, safflower oil (hybrid), sunflower oil (hybrid) |

**Table 10: Fats in Foods**

**Trans fats** are produced when a liquid oil is processed into a solid fat. The manufacturing process is called hydrogenation, or partial hydrogenation, and trans fats are an unnatural by-product. Partially-hydrogenated vegetable oils are considered especially unhealthy, because of the resulting trans-fatty acids and the added hydrogen saturation. Research indicates that trans fats are even worse than saturated fats because they not only raise bad LDL cholesterol but also lower good HDL cholesterol. Eliminating foods containing partially-hydrogenated oils from your diet is vital to good health.

In summary, it is becoming increasingly clear that saturated and trans fats, increase the risk for certain diseases while monounsaturated and polyunsaturated fats, lower the risk. The key is not to eliminate fat from your diet but to substitute good fats for bad fats, and at the same time try to reduce the total amount of fat consumed because all fats are very high in calories. The current scientific thinking regarding fat consumption is as follows:

**1)** Try to limit the total fat you eat to no more than 30 percent of your caloric intake.

**2)** Do not consume foods containing partially-hydrogenated vegetable oil because they are high in trans fats. This includes commercially prepared baked goods, snack foods, and processed foods, including fast foods. To be on the safe-side, assume these food products contain trans fats unless labeled otherwise.

**3)** Limit saturated fats, i.e., any fat of animal origin, to 10 percent of your caloric intake. Have meat less often, and when serving meat use lean cuts and trim the fat. Eat fish and poultry (white meat, without the skin) more frequently. Use fat-free or low-fat-milk dairy products in place of whole-milk dairy products. (Coconut and palm oil should also be avoided because they are saturated fats.)

**4)** When consuming fat, choose foods containing monounsaturated fats like olive oil and canola oil, and foods rich in polyunsaturated omega-6 and omega-3 fatty acids.

**5)** Try to balance your intake essential fatty acids by eating more omega-3 fatty acids, found in walnuts, tofu, certain seeds and oily fish such as salmon, sardines and tuna.

## Vitamins and Minerals

The following is a listing of vitamins and minerals complete with a brief discussion of their function in your body, what foods supply the particular micronutrient, and the Recommended Dietary Allowance (RDA) - which is a reference number developed by the United States Food and Drug Administration to help consumers determine how much of a specific micronutrient a food contains. Summaries of the RDAs for vitamins and minerals are shown in Table 11a, 11b, 12a and 12b on pages 51, 52, 55 and 56. Notice that RDAs are frequently gender and age dependent.

Because of the rapid expansion of scientific knowledge regarding the role of micronutrients in human health, the U.S. Food and Drug Administration, in partnership with Health Canada, periodically assesses and updates the recommended Daily Values. The following contains the recommended RDAs as of April 2006 for the vitamins and minerals discussed.

**Vitamin A** is a collection of fat-soluble compounds that play an important role in vision, bone growth, reproduction, cell division, and help prevent or fight off infections. Vitamin A also promotes healthy surface linings of the eyes, respiratory, urinary, and intestinal tracts, and also helps maintain the integrity of skin and mucous membranes. Using the long-established International Unit (IU) measure for the recommended dietary allowance (RDA), adult men and women need 3,000 and 2,330 IU (as retinol) per day respectively. However, the new RDA measure for vitamin A is the microgram (mcg), which translates for men and women as 900 and 700 mcg per day. Foods rich in vitamin A are orange-colored vegetables such as carrots, sweet potatoes and pumpkin; dark-green-leafy vegetables like spinach, collards and romaine lettuce; and orange-colored fruits such as mango, cantaloupe and apricots; and red peppers and tomatoes. One medium-size carrot supplies approximately 270 percent of your RDA.

**Vitamin D** is a fat-soluble vitamin. Briefly, vitamin D is important in assisting the absorption of calcium, in forming strong bones and teeth and preventing deficiency diseases such as rickets and osteomalacia. For most adults, an adequate intake of vitamin D is 200 to 600 IU (which is equivalent to 5 to 15 mcg per day). In addition, your body can make vitamin D after exposure to sunshine. Good food sources include salt-water fish such as herring, salmon, sardines and fish-liver oils, as well as fortified milk and cereals. Small quantities are also found in egg yokes, veal and beef. An eight-ounce glass of fortified milk supplies about 25 percent of your daily needs.

**Vitamin E** is a fat-soluble vitamin that is a powerful antioxidant and acts to protect cells against the effects of free radicals. Research is underway to determine if vitamin E, through its ability to limit the production of free radicals, might help prevent or delay the development of cardiovascular disease and some cancers. For adults, the RDA for vitamin E is 22.5 IU (as d-alpha-tocopherol) which is equal to 15 mcg per day. Foods rich in vitamin E are vegetable oils, nuts, seeds, milk fat, egg yolks, liver, dark-green-leafy vegetables, and whole-grain foods. Approximately 12 almonds provide 100 percent of RDA for vitamin E.

| Vitamin | Ages | | | |
|---|---|---|---|---|
| | 19-30 | 31-50 | 51-70 | 70+ |
| A (mcg) | 900 | 900 | 900 | 900 |
| D (mcg) | 5 | 5 | 10 | 15 |
| E (mcg) | 15 | 15 | 15 | 15 |
| K (mcg) | 120 | 120 | 120 | 120 |
| C (mg) | 90 | 90 | 90 | 90 |
| $B_1$ (mg) | 1.2 | 1.2 | 1.2 | 1.2 |
| $B_2$ (mg) | 1.3 | 1.3 | 1.3 | 1.3 |
| $B_3$ (mg) | 16 | 16 | 16 | 16 |
| $B_5$ (mg) | 5 | 5 | 5 | 5 |
| $B_6$ (mg) | 1.3 | 1.3 | 1.7 | 1.7 |
| $B_7$ (mcg) | 30 | 30 | 30 | 30 |
| $B_9$ (mcg) | 400 | 400 | 400 | 400 |
| $B_{12}$ (mcg) | 2.4 | 2.4 | 2.4 | 2.4 |

**Table 11a: Vitamin RDA for Men**

Values for vitamins D, K, $B_5$ and $B_7$ are Adequate Intake.  mcg = micrograms per day mg = milligrams per day.

**Vitamin K** is another fat-soluble vitamin, and is known as the clotting vitamin because without it blood would not clot. Some studies also indicate that it helps maintain strong bones in the elderly. Adequate intake of vitamin K for men is 120 mcg per day and for women 90 mcg per day.  Food sources are dark-green-leafy vegetables, soybean, cottonseed, canola, and olive oil. People who eat these foods as part of a balanced diet should easily get enough vitamin K.

**Vitamin C** is a water-soluble, antioxidant vitamin.  It is important in forming collagen, a protein that gives structure to bones, cartilage, muscle, and blood vessels. Vitamin C also aids in the absorption of iron, and helps maintain capillaries, bones, and teeth. The RDA for vitamin C is 90 milligrams (mg) per day for men and 75 mg per day for women. Foods rich in vitamin C are citrus fruits and juices, kiwifruit, strawberries, cantaloupe, broccoli, peppers, tomatoes, cabbage potatoes, and dark-green-leafy vegetables. A six-ounce glass of orange juice supplies 100 percent of a man's RDA.

| Vitamin | Ages | | | | | |
|---|---|---|---|---|---|---|
| | 19-30 | 31-50 | 51-70 | 70+ | Preg | Lact |
| A (mcg) | 700 | 700 | 700 | 700 | 770 | 1300 |
| D (mcg) | 5 | 5 | 10 | 15 | 5 | 5 |
| E (mcg) | 15 | 15 | 15 | 15 | 15 | 19 |
| K (mcg) | 90 | 90 | 90 | 90 | 90 | 90 |
| C (mg) | 75 | 75 | 75 | 75 | 85 | 120 |
| $B_1$ (mg) | 1.1 | 1.1 | 1.1 | 1.1 | 1.4 | 1.4 |
| $B_2$ (mg) | 1.1 | 1.1 | 1.1 | 1.1 | 1.4 | 1.6 |
| $B_3$ (mg) | 14 | 14 | 14 | 14 | 18 | 17 |
| $B_5$ (mg) | 5 | 5 | 5 | 5 | 6 | 7 |
| $B_6$ (mg) | 1.3 | 1.3 | 1.5 | 1.5 | 1.9 | 2.0 |
| $B_7$ (mcg) | 30 | 30 | 30 | 30 | 30 | 35 |
| $B_9$ (mcg) | 400 | 400 | 400 | 400 | 600 | 500 |
| $B_{12}$ (mcg) | 2.4 | 2.4 | 2.4 | 2.4 | 2.6 | 2.8 |

**Table 11b: Vitamin RDA for Women**
Values for vitamins D, K, $B_5$ and $B_7$ are Adequate Intake. Preg = pregnant  Lact = lactating  mcg = micrograms per day  mg = milligrams per day.

**Vitamin B** is actually a complex of different water-soluble vitamins that often exist in the same foods. They perform an important role in our metabolism, in maintaining muscle tone along our digestive tract and in the health of our nervous system, skin, hair, eyes, mouth, and liver. he B complex vitamins are: vitamin $B_1$ (thiamine), vitamin $B_2$ (riboflavin), vitamin $B_3$ (niacin), vitamin $B_5$ (pantothenic acid), vitamin $B_6$ (pyridoxine), vitamin $B_7$ (biotin), vitamin $B_9$ (folic acid), and vitamin $B_{12}$ (cyanocobalamin). Many cereals are fortified with all the B vitamins.

Depending on the brand, one serving of a fortified cereal provides from 25 to 100 percent of the RDA for all the B vitamins (except vitamin $B_7$ biotin).

**Vitamin $B_1$ (thiamine)** plays a vital role in the proper operation of your nervous system. Your body also needs $B_1$ to convert carbohydrates into sugar and then energy. The RDA for men is 1.2 mg per day and 1.1 mg per day for women. Vitamin $B_1$ is found in meat, wheat germ, whole-grains cereals and breads, in enriched cereals and breads, in beans, nuts and seeds, and in dark-green-leafy vegetables.

**Vitamin $B_2$ (riboflavin)** also has a crucial role in certain metabolic reactions, particularly the conversion of carbohydrates into energy. Riboflavin is also an important antioxidant. he RDA is 1.3 mg per day for men and 1.1 mg per day for women. he best sources of riboflavin are brewer's yeast, almonds, organ meats, whole grains, wheat germ, wild rice, mushrooms, soybeans, milk, yogurt, eggs, broccoli, and spinach. In addition, flour and cereals are often fortified with riboflavin.

**Vitamin $B_3$ (niacin)** helps clear toxic and harmful chemicals from your body. It also assists in the production of various hormones. Niacin improves your circulation and reduces blood cholesterol levels. The RDA is 16 mg per day for men and 14 mg per day for women. Foods containing significant amounts of niacin are liver, meat, poultry, fish, whole-grains and nuts.

**Vitamin $B_5$ (pantothenic acid)** is necessary for a variety of life-sustaining tasks such as generating energy from food, synthesizing essential fats, and the function of your adrenal glands. Adequate intake of vitamin $B_5$ for adults is 5 mg per day. Good sources include organ meats, eggs, fish and shellfish, poultry, soybeans, beans, dairy foods, avocado, and mushrooms.

**Vitamin $B_6$ (pyridoxine)** is needed for protein and red-blood cell metabolism. Your body also requires vitamin $B_6$ to make hemoglobin. For men and women up to 50 years old, the RDA is 1.3 mg per day. After 50, the RDA increases to 1.7 mg per day for men and 1.5 mg for women. Vitamin $B_6$ is found in a wide variety of foods including fortified cereals, beans, meat, poultry, fish, and some fruits and vegetables.

**Vitamin $B_7$ (biotin)** functions as a coenzyme in the synthesis of fat, glycogen and amino acids. An adequate intake of biotin is 30 mcg per day. A varied diet should provide enough biotin for most people. Liver, yeast and egg yokes are particularly rich food sources. It is also found in smaller amounts in fruit, meat and cheese.

**Vitamin B$_9$ (folate or folic acid)** helps produce and maintain new cells which is particularly important during periods of rapid cell division and growth such as in infancy and during pregnancy. Folate is needed to make DNA and RNA, the building blocks of cells. It is also thought to prevent DNA changes that may lead to cancer. For most adults, the RDA of folate is 400 mcg per day. Of course, woman who are expecting or nursing need more folate. Cooked dry beans and peas, peanuts, oranges, dark-green-leafy vegetables and green peas are folate-rich foods.

**Vitamin B$_{12}$ (cyanocobalamin)** enables your body to manufacture healthy red-blood cells. It also assists in the transmission of electrical signals between nerve cells. The recommended dietary allowance is 2.4 mcg per day. Vitamin B$_{12}$ is found in fortified cereals, meat, fish and poultry.

**Calcium** is a mineral with several important functions. Most of the calcium in your body is used to support the structure of your bones and teeth. A small amount of calcium is in your blood, muscle, and the fluid between your cells. Calcium is also needed for muscle contraction, blood vessel contraction and expansion, the secretion of hormones and enzymes, and sending messages through the nervous system. For most adults, adequate intake is 1,000 mg per day. Foods rich in calcium are milk, yogurt, natural cheeses (such as cheddar, Swiss and mozzarella), canned fish with soft bones such as salmon and sardines, and dark-green-leafy vegetables. Eight ounces of milk (whole or skim) contains 30 percent of your RDA.

**Chromium** is important in the metabolism of fats and carbohydrates and in controlling blood sugar levels. It is an activator of several enzymes needed to drive numerous chemical reactions necessary to life. For men and women up to 50 years old, an adequate intake of chromium is 35 and 25 mcg per day respectively. After 50, the suggested adequate intake drops to 30 mcg per day for men and 20 for women. Whole grains, ready-to-eat bran cereals, seafood, green beans, broccoli, prunes, nuts, peanut butter, and potatoes are rich in chromium. One-half cup of chopped broccoli provides about 35 percent of your chromium RDA.

| Mineral | Ages | | | |
|---|---|---|---|---|
| | 19-30 | 31-50 | 51-70 | 70+ |
| **Calcium** (mg) | 1000 | 1000 | 1200 | 1200 |
| **Chromium** (mcg) | 35 | 35 | 30 | 30 |
| **Copper** (mcg) | 900 | 900 | 900 | 900 |
| **Fluoride** (mg) | 4 | 4 | 4 | 4 |
| **Iodine** (mcg) | 150 | 150 | 150 | 150 |
| **Iron** (mg) | 8 | 8 | 8 | 8 |
| **Magnesium** (mg) | 400 | 420 | 420 | 420 |
| **Manganese** (mg) | 2.3 | 2.3 | 2.3 | 2.3 |
| **Molybdenum** (mcg) | 45 | 45 | 45 | 45 |
| **Phosphorus** (mg) | 700 | 700 | 700 | 700 |
| **Potassium** (mg) | 4700 | 4700 | 4700 | 4700 |
| **Selenium** (mcg) | 55 | 55 | 55 | 55 |
| **Zinc** (mg) | 11 | 11 | 11 | 11 |

**Table 12a: Mineral RDA for Men**

Values for calcium, chromium, fluoride & manganese are Adequate Intake. mcg = micrograms per day  mg = milligrams per day

**Iodine** is a basic component of the thyroid hormone that regulates your metabolic rate. Lack of iodine can cause a number of physical and mental abnormalities. RDA for adult men and women is 150 mcg per day. Iodized salt, sea food and plants grown in iodine-rich soil are good sources of iodine. A three-ounce serving of cooked haddock contains about 125 mcg of iodine.

**Iron** is an important mineral that aids the transport of oxygen in your body and is also needed for the regulation of cell growth. An iron deficiency limits oxygen delivery to cells, resulting in fatigue and decreased immunity. The RDA for iron is 8 mg per day for men and 18

| Mineral | Ages | | | | | |
|---|---|---|---|---|---|---|
| | 19-30 | 31-50 | 51-70 | 70+ | Preg | Lact |
| Calcium (mg) | 1000 | 1000 | 1200 | 1200 | 1000 | 1000 |
| Chromium (mcg) | 25 | 25 | 20 | 20 | 30 | 45 |
| Copper (mcg) | 900 | 900 | 900 | 900 | 1000 | 1300 |
| Fluoride (mg) | 3 | 3 | 3 | 3 | 3 | 3 |
| Iodine (mcg) | 150 | 150 | 150 | 150 | 220 | 290 |
| Iron (mg) | 18 | 18 | 8 | 8 | 27 | 9 |
| Magnesium (mg) | 310 | 320 | 320 | 320 | 355 | 315 |
| Manganese (mg) | 1.8 | 1.8 | 1.8 | 1.8 | 2.0 | 2.6 |
| Molybdenum (mcg) | 45 | 45 | 45 | 45 | 50 | 50 |
| Phosphorus (mg) | 700 | 700 | 700 | 700 | 700 | 700 |
| Potassium (mg) | 4700 | 4700 | 4700 | 4700 | 4700 | 5100 |
| Selenium (mcg) | 55 | 55 | 55 | 55 | 60 | 70 |
| Zinc (mg) | 8 | 8 | 8 | 8 | 8 | 8 |

**Table 12b: Mineral RDA for Women**
Preg = pregnant   Lact = lactating  mcg = micrograms per day  mg = milligrams per day.
Values for calcium, chromium, fluoride & manganese are Adequate Intake.

mg per day for pre-menopausal women. Foods rich in iron are shrimp, clams, mussels, oysters, sardines, lean meats (especially beef), organ meats, turkey (dark meat), spinach, cooked dry beans, peas, lentils, and whole-grain breads and cereals. Three ounces of beef liver has approximately 50 percent of your iron RDA, and fortified cereals can provide from 50 to 100 percent of your RDA.

**Magnesium** is needed for hundreds of biochemical reactions in your body. It helps maintain normal muscle and nerve function, keeps heart rhythm steady, supports a healthy immune system, and keeps bones strong. The RDA is 420 mg per day for men and 320 for women. Dark-green-leafy vegetables, fish, some beans and peas, nuts and seeds, and whole grains are good sources of magnesium. One-half cup of cooked spinach has 75 mg of magnesium.

**Phosphorus** in combination with calcium is necessary for the formation of bones and teeth. Phosphorus is also involved in the metabolism of fats, carbohydrates and proteins, and in the effective utilization of many of the B vitamins. The RDA for adults is 700 mg per day. Rich sources of phosphorus are dairy products, meat, and fish. Phosphorus is also present in most soft drinks. Generally, a diet that provides adequate amounts of calcium and protein also provides a sufficient amount of phosphorus.

**Potassium** is involved in proper nerve function, muscle control and blood pressure regulation. (People engaged in vigorous exercise may need more potassium to replace that lost during exercise.) Low potassium levels can cause muscle cramping and cardiovascular irregularities. Adequate intake for men and women is 4,700 mg per day. Potassium-rich foods include baked white or sweet potatoes, cooked leafy greens, winter (orange) squash, bananas, oranges, dried fruits (such as apricots and prunes), and cooked dry beans and lentils. A medium-size baked potato contains about 600 mg of potassium.

**Selenium** is an essential trace element that assists enzymes involved in antioxidant protection and thyroid hormone metabolism. The RDA is 55 mcg per day for men and women. The most important sources in American diets are meats, fish and grains. Three ounces of cooked cod provide about 32 mcg of selenium.

**Zinc** is an essential mineral that stimulates the activity of approximately 100 enzymes that promote biochemical reactions in your body. Zinc supports a healthy immune system needed for wound healing, and helps maintain your sense of taste and smell. The RDA for zinc is 11 mg per day for men and 8 mg per day for women. Oysters contain more zinc per serving than any other food. Other good sources are red meat, poultry, beans, nuts, certain seafood, whole grains, dairy products and fortified breakfast cereals which can provide from 50 to 100 percent of your RDA.

# Guidelines for Healthy Eating

No single food can supply all the nutrients you need in the amounts you need. The most important factors in nutrition are variety, variety, variety! **Variety is the key to a nutritious diet**. As a means of setting strategies for food selection, the U.S. Department of Health and Human Services and the Department of Agriculture issue Dietary Guidelines every five years. The latest Dietary Guidelines recommend the following:

– **Make Half your Plate Fruits and Vegetables:** Eat red, orange, and dark-green vegetables, such as tomatoes, sweet potatoes, and broccoli. Eat fruit, vegetables, or unsalted nuts as snacks.

– **Switch to Skim or 1% Milk:** Both have the same amount of calcium and other essential nutrients as whole milk, but less fat and calories. If lactose intolerant, try calcium-fortified soy products as an alternative to dairy foods.

– **Make at least Half your Grains Whole:** Choose 100% wholegrain cereals, breads, crackers, rice, and pasta. Check the ingredients list on food packages to find whole-grain foods.

– **Vary your Protein Food choices:** Twice a week, make seafood the protein on your plate. Eat beans, a natural source of fiber and protein. Keep meat and poultry portions small & lean.

– **Choose Foods and Drinks with little or No Added Sugars:** Drink water instead of sugary drinks. Select fruit for dessert. Eat sugary desserts less often. Choose 100% fruit juice instead of fruit-flavored drinks.

– **Look Out for Salt (sodium) in Foods you Buy:** Compare sodium in foods like soup, bread, and frozen meals and choose the foods with lower numbers. Add spices or herbs to season food without adding salt.

– **Eat Fewer Foods that are High in Solid Fats:** Make major sources of saturated fats – such as cakes, cookies, ice cream, pizza, cheese, sausages, and hot dogs – occasional choices, not everyday foods. Select lean cuts of meats or poultry and fat-free or low-fat milk, yogurt, and cheese. Switch from solid fats to oils when preparing food.

– **To Maintain a Healthy Weight:** Basically enjoy your food, but eat less. Stay within your personal calorie limit. (Note that caloric needs will be covered in a later chapter.) Think before you eat: Is it worth the calories? Avoid oversized portions. Use a smaller plate, bowl, and glass. Stop eating when you are satisfied, not full.

– **Know your personal Daily Calorie Limit:** Keep that calorie number in mind when deciding what to eat. ( Again, caloric needs will be covered in a later chapter.) Use a food log to keep track of how much you eat.

– **When Eating out Check posted Calorie Amounts:** Choose lower calorie menu options. Select dishes that include vegetables, fruits, and/or whole grains. Order a smaller portion or share when eating out. Cook more often at home, where you are in control of what's in your food.

– **If you Drink Alcoholic beverages, do so Sensibly:** Limit should be 1 drink a day for women or to 2 drinks a day for men.

## Basic Food Groups

In this section we describe the various food groups, indicate what constitutes a serving size, and focus on the best foods within each group. (The foods in **bold font** are generally the most nutrient-dense foods – the best of the best.)

**Fruit Group**: Includes fresh, frozen, canned and dried fruits and fruit juices. Usually, a serving is 1 cup. A serving from the fruit group consists of 1 cup of fresh, frozen or canned fruit, or 1 cup of 100 percent fruit juice, or ½ cup of dried fruit. This group can be divided further into citrus fruits, berries and grapes, and other fruits.

**Citrus fruits**: There are many excellent citrus choices including **oranges, grapefruit, lemons, limes, kiwifruit and kumquats**. All are low calorie foods that contain a negligible amount of fat and cholesterol, are high in vitamin C, and most have significant amounts of vitamin A, potassium and dietary fiber.

**Berries & grapes**: Among the fruits in this grouping are **blackberries, blueberries, raspberries, strawberries, cranberries, gooseberries, purple grapes, black currents, raisins, and cherries**. Every fresh berry and grape is low calorie, with no fat or cholesterol, and all have small amounts of multiple micronutrients and a fair amount of dietary fiber. (Strawberries are also rich in vitamin C.) Some researchers claim that the blue and black-colored berries are packed with more disease-fighting antioxidants than any other fruit or vegetable. Of course, dark-red and purple grape contain the phytonutrient flavonol, the same antioxidant believed to give red wine its heart-protecting benefits.

**Other fruits**: This large subgroup includes a number of healthy foods such as **apples, apricots, bananas, cantaloupe, figs, mangos, papayas, peaches, pears, pineapples, plums, prunes and watermelon**. Again, most are low calorie, contain no fat or cholesterol, and are loaded with vitamins, minerals and phytonutrients. In addition, apples, apricots, figs, peaches, pears, pineapples, plums, prunes are good sources of dietary fiber. Cantaloupe is also high in vitamin C and watermelon contains the phytonutrient lycopene.

**Vegetable Group**: Includes fresh, frozen, dried and canned vegetables and vegetable juices. In general, 1 cup from the vegetable group consists of 1 cup of raw or cooked vegetables or vegetable juice, or 2 cups of raw-leafy greens. This group can be broken down further into dark-green-leafy vegetables, orange-colored vegetables, starchy vegetables and other vegetables.

**Dark-green-leafy vegetables**: Every food in this category (which includes **bok choy, collard greens, kale, mustard greens, romaine lettuce, spinach, Swiss chard and turnip greens**) is low calorie with no fat or cholesterol, and is packed with micronutrients, especially vitamins A and C, calcium, iron, potassium and folate, as well as dietary fiber.

**Orange-colored vegetables**: The best in this subgroup are **carrots, orange-bell peppers, pumpkin, sweet potatoes, yams and winter squash**. All have negligible fat and cholesterol and are high in vitamin A, potassium and dietary fiber.

**Starchy vegetables**: This grouping overlaps somewhat with the orange-colored vegetable subgroup and the grains group. Among the foods included are **white potatoes, sweet potatoes, yams, yellow corn, and brown rice**. These vegetables are generally high in complex carbohydrates, B vitamins, potassium and dietary fiber.

**Other vegetables:** This extensive category contains **asparagus, broccoli, Brussels sprouts, cabbage, cauliflower, celery, cucumber, fennel, green beans, parsley, and summer squash**. The preceding are low calorie foods that contain a negligible amount of fat and cholesterol, and most have significant amounts of vitamins A and C, potassium, calcium, iron, other micronutrients and dietary fiber. Also in this category are **eggplant, garlic, leeks, onions and mushrooms** which contain few calories, no cholesterol, and important amounts of potassium, calcium, iron and other micronutrients, as well as dietary fiber. **Red peppers and tomatoes** are low-calorie vegetables with no cholesterol that are loaded with vitamins A and C, iron and dietary fiber. Tomatoes also contain the phytonutrient lycopene. **Avocado and olives** contain some beneficial monounsaturated and polyunsaturated fat, but no cholesterol. Avocados are relatively high in potassium and vitamin A, while olives have significant amounts of iron and calcium.

**Grains Group**: Includes all foods made from wheat, rice, oats, cornmeal and barley, such as bread, pasta, oatmeal, breakfast cereals and grits. Generally, 1 ounce from the grains group consists of 1 thin slice of bread, or 1 cup of ready-to-eat cereal, or ½ cup of cooked rice, pasta or cooked cereal. <u>At least half of the grains eaten should be whole grains.</u>

Grains are the seeds of varied grasses grown for food. The outermost layer of the grain is an inedible husk, called chaff. The next layer is the bran, a protective coating rich in fiber. When this layer is removed, the product is described as pearled or polished. Inside the bran is the endosperm (the starchy part of a grain) and the germ, the part highest in nutrients (e.g., wheat germ). Whole grains have all these components intact. Refined grains have the husk, bran, and germ removed. Many foods are a mixture of whole and refined grains. Check the ingredient list for the words "whole grain" or "whole wheat" to determine if a food is made from a whole grain. In the United States, to be labeled "whole grain" a food must contain more than 51 percent whole grain by weight.

**Whole grains** include: **barley, buckwheat, bulgur, corn, millet, oats, brown rice, rye, wheat and wild rice**. Some whole-grain foods are: **whole-wheat bread, whole-grain ready-to-eat cereal, whole-wheat crackers, oatmeal, popcorn, whole-wheat pasta**, and whole barley (in beef-barley soup). All grains are low in fat and contain no cholesterol. Whole grains are good sources of complex carbohydrates and dietary fiber, as well as several B vitamins (thiamin, riboflavin, niacin, and folate), vitamin E, and minerals (iron, magnesium, and selenium).

**Meats, Beans (and nuts) Group**: Generally, 1 ounce equivalent from this group consists of 1 ounce of lean meat, poultry, or fish, or 1 egg, or 1 tablespoon of peanut butter, or ¼ cup cooked dry beans, or ½ cup of nuts or seeds. This group can be divided further into subgroups consisting of meat and foul, fish, eggs, beans, and nuts and seeds.

**Meat and Foul**: **Skinless white-meat chicken and turkey** are relatively low calorie, low fat, low cholesterol foods that are powerful sources of high-quality protein, vitamin $B_6$, riboflavin, niacin, phosphorus and potassium. Most meats, even **lean meats**, are higher in fat and calories than chicken and turkey, but meats do provide high-quality protein and some important nutrients such as iron and B-vitamins.

**Fish:** Most fish are good choices including **cod, halibut, herring, mackerel, salmon, sardines, scallops, shrimp, snapper, trout and tuna.** Nearly all fish contain high levels of essential-fatty acids. (Oily cold-water fish such as wild salmon, sardines, herring, mackerel and tuna are high in omega-3 essential-fatty acid. Trout also has comparatively high omega-3 content.) All fish are relatively low-calorie foods and are good sources of the fat-soluble vitamins A and D. (Fish-liver oils have high levels of fat soluble vitamins, and have been used as dietary supplements for many years.) Nutritionally, seafood is better known for its dietary minerals than for its vitamins. This is because some minerals in fish, such as iodine and selenium, are not available at the same levels in most other non-marine foods. Fish are also a good source of iron and potassium.

There is, however, a downside to eating fish. Some fish are contaminated with mercury, PCBs, dioxins and other environmental pollutants. Mercury is a toxic heavy metal that can accumulate in certain fish species. Large predatory fish such as shark, swordfish, king mackerel and tilefish have the highest concentration of mercury and other environmental contaminates. Canned white albacore tuna, a commonly eaten fish, contains higher levels of mercury than canned light tuna . The U.S. Food and Drug Administration advises adults to eat no more than six ounces of high-mercury fish per week.

PCBs are potential human carcinogens that find their way into fresh waters and oceans where they are absorbed by fish. A recent study reported that PCB levels in farmed salmon, especially those in from Europe, were about seven times higher than in wild salmon.

For further information about the safety of fish you catch locally, have your client visit the U.S. Environmental Protection Agency's Fish Advisory website or contact your state or local health department. If no advice is available, eat no more than six ounces per week of fish caught from local waters and do not consume any other fish that week.

According to the University of Michigan Integrative Medicine Department, pregnant and nursing women, and young children, should avoid shark, swordfish, king mackerel and tilefish, and strictly limit the amount of other contaminated fish consumed.

**Eggs:** Current dietary guidelines and the latest research concerning egg consumption appear to be at odds. On the one hand, because a typical egg yoke contains saturated fat and 300 mg of cholesterol, the latest dietary guidelines recommend that egg yolks and whole eggs be used in moderation (up to one egg per day), but that egg whites and most egg substitutes can be used freely since they contain no cholesterol and little or no fat.

On the other hand, others argue that if judged as a whole food and not simply as a source of cholesterol, positives such as the fact that eggs are low calorie, are loaded with high-quality protein, are a good source of vitamin E, etcetera, are apparent. Moreover, researchers at the Harvard Medical School studied egg consumption among 120,000 nurses and other health professionals with normal cholesterol levels and reported no link between eating eggs and heart disease or stroke.

Some medical researchers advise that, if one is at low risk (i.e., does not smoke, exercises regularly, eats a healthy diet and has no family history of heart disease or stroke) and chooses to begin eating eggs, they should have a blood test four to six weeks after they start eating eggs to determine the impact on their total and LDL cholesterol. Based on the test results, your client and her doctor can decide – yes or no to her eating more eggs.

**Beans:** Among the foods in this important subgroup are **black beans, cannelloni beans, dried peas, fava beans, garbanzo beans, red kidney beans, lentils, lima beans, navy beans, and pinto beans**. All beans are inexpensive, low-fat, plant-protein-rich foods that are good sources of B vitamins, potassium, iron, dietary fiber and isoflavones (important phytonutrients).

**Nuts and Seeds:** This category consists of **almonds, cashews, hazelnuts, peanuts, pecans, pistachio nuts, walnuts, flaxseed, pumpkin seeds, sesame seeds, sunflower seeds**, and others. Because nuts and seeds contain significant amounts of essential-fatty acids, they are comparatively high-calorie foods. Most nuts and seeds have a good amount of dietary fiber, vitamin E, potassium, iron and folate. Almonds, cashews, peanuts, and pine nuts contain a significant quantity of plant protein and essential-fatty acids. Walnuts, flaxseed and pumpkin seeds are important sources of plant-based omega-3 fatty acids.

**Soy:** The soybean is the most widely grown legume. Healthful soy foods such as **tofu, soy nuts, soymilk, soybean oil, and soy protein** are made from soybeans. All contain a significant amount of plant-based complete protein and omega-3 fatty acid as well as vitamin E, potassium, iron and folate. Soy nuts are also high in dietary fiber.

Soybeans, tofu, and other soy-based foods are an excellent alternative to red meat. But there are some suspected dangers from too much soy. So advise your client not to overdo it. The Harvard University School of Public Health recommends two to four servings of soy foods per week as a good goal. Furthermore, they caution adults not to take supplements that contain concentrated soy protein or soy extracts, such as isoflavones.

**Milk Group:** Includes liquid milk and all products and foods made from milk such yogurt and cheese. (Foods that have little or no calcium such as cream, butter and cream cheese are not in this group.) In general, 1 cup from the milk group consists of 1 cup of milk or yogurt, or 1½ ounces of natural cheese, or 2 ounces of processed cheese.

**Milk, yogurt and natural cheeses** are high in calcium and protein. **Milk** is also often fortified with vitamin D. In addition to calcium and protein, **yogurt** is a particularly wholesome food providing live active bacteria cultures which promote gastrointestinal health. Most choices in this group should be fat free or low fat.

**Oils Group:** Includes vegetable oils and foods such as **nuts, olives, oily fish, avocados**, mayonnaise, soft margarine and some salad dressings. You should limit the intake of saturated fats – that is any fat of animal origin.

The oils group overlaps somewhat with many of the others. Liquid oils, however, are unique to this group. **Corn oil, flaxseed oil, safflower oil, sesame oil, soybean oil and sunflower oil** are polyunsaturated; whereas, **canola oil, olive oil and peanut oil** are monounsaturated. All these oils are high in calories and essential-fatty acids. Essential-fatty acids promote absorption of the fat-soluble vitamins A, D, E, and K. Flaxseed, canola and soybean oil contain omega-3 fatty acids. (Note, when purchasing olive oil, choose an oil that is labeled "extra-virgin" or "virgin." Virgin olive oils are produced from the first pressing of the olives, are unrefined and as a result are more healthful.)

## Vitamin/Mineral Supplements

Even though most adults can get all the vitamins and minerals they need by merely consuming a variety of nutritious foods (from the fruit group, the vegetable group, the grains group, the meat and beans group, the milk group, and the oils group), **many physicians recommend a daily multi-vitamin/mineral supplement as a kind of insurance policy**.

Be aware that some micronutrients, such as the fat-soluble vitamin A, can be harmful if taken in large quantities. To be safe your multi-vitamin/mineral supplement should contain no more than 100 percent of the recommended dietary allowance (RDA) for each vitamin or mineral. Generally, you don't need the high doses in multi-vitamin/mineral supplements labeled "therapeutic" or "extra-strength." There may be medical reasons for taking larger amounts of a vitamin or mineral than the RDA provides, but check with your doctor first. For example, a physician may advise a pregnant woman to take an iron supplement, and women who could become pregnant to take folic acid in addition to consuming folate-rich foods to reduce the risk of some serious birth defects. Adults over age 50 and vegetarians who do not eat animal foods may be advised to get their vitamin $B_{12}$ from a supplement or from fortified foods. Women with little exposure to sunlight may need a vitamin D supplement, and individuals who seldom eat dairy products or other rich sources of calcium may need to take a calcium supplement.

Dietary supplement choices include not only vitamins and minerals, but also herbal products and many other widely available substances. Herbal products, however, usually provide only small amounts of vitamins and minerals and their health value is currently being studied.

## You Need Fiber

Fiber is an important part of a healthy diet. **You need to consume fiber to assist your digestive system**. According to the Harvard University School of Public Health, adequate fiber intake reduces the risk of developing various conditions, including heart disease, diabetes, diverticular disease, and constipation.

Three fibers that are eaten on a regular basis are cellulose, hemicellulose and pectin. Hemicellulose is found in the hulls of different grains like wheat; e.g., wheat bran is hemicellulose. Cellulose is the structural component of plants, and gives vegetables their familiar shape. Pectin is found most often in fruits, is soluble in water but non-digestible, and is usually referred to as "water-soluble fiber." The best fiber sources are:
- Whole-grain breads, whole-grain cereals, whole-wheat pasta and brown rice contain a great deal of hemicellulose fiber.
- Fruits are pectin rich (the water-soluble fiber). The skin on fruits are loaded with phytonutrients and fiber. So do not peal an apple. Eat it with

the skin on and get a fiber and nutrient boost.

- Most berries (such as bilberries, raspberries) have even more fiber than a comparable weight of most other fruit selections.

- Vegetables have lots of cellulose fiber. Again the skin is particularly high in fiber. When you eat a baked potato, eat it skin and all – everything – everything that is except the butter or sour cream.

- Peas and beans are high fiber foods that are also a complete protein when eaten with a whole grain food, or nuts, or seeds.

- Nuts and seeds add fiber to your diet.

When you eat fiber, in any of its forms, it simply passes straight through, untouched by but aiding your digestive system. Zero calories absorbed!

**Adults should get a least 20 to 35 grams of dietary fiber per day**. How much fiber is in the foods you eat? An apple has 3 grams of fiber, a tangerine has 2 grams, ½ cup cabbage contains 2 grams, a tomato has 2 grams, ½ cup broccoli has 1 gram, ½ cup of lima beans contains 4 grams, 1 cup of brown rice has 3 grams, 1 cup of whole-wheat cereal holds 3 grams and 1 slice of whole-wheat bread contains 2 grams of fiber.

## Drink Lots of Water

The average adult female body is about 52 percent water, while the average adult male is approximately 63 percent water. If you are average, everyday you lose about 10 cups of water when you breathe, perspire, and excrete waste. Because water is needed for almost every biochemical and physiologic process in your body, to maintain your body's water balance you must replace this lost water. (The water in your body is said to be balanced, when your water intake from all sources equals your loss of water.)

Typically, the food you eat every day contains about 3 cups of mostly concealed water. When you metabolize the food you eat, you create another cup of water. That leaves about six cups that must be replaced by the liquids you drink – even more when you exercise. It appears, therefore, that the long-established wisdom advocating that you drink eight glasses of water per day (or any other healthy beverage such as tea or fruit juice) is not far from the mark.

## Use Salt Sparingly

Sodium and sodium chloride (salt) normally occur in small quantities in many natural foods. Salt and sodium-containing ingredients are also frequently found in high amounts in processed foods, such as canned soup and baked goods.  People also add salt during food preparation and to the food they eat.  Although sodium plays an important role in your body, many studies have demonstrated that high sodium intake is also associated with high blood pressure.  In your body, sodium retains water expanding blood volume which in turn raises blood pressure.  Moreover, although some questions remain, evidence suggests that many adults who are predisposed to high blood pressure (for example having a parent who has high blood pressure) can reduce their chances of developing high blood pressure by consuming less sodium.

Most Americans consume too much sodium.  The U.S. Department of Health and Human Services and the Department of Agriculture Dietary Guidelines recommend that healthy adults **limit sodium intake to 2,400 mg per day.**  (Note that one level teaspoon of salt contains about 2,300 mg of sodium.)  Individuals who have high blood pressure and are also salt sensitive are frequently advised to limit their sodium intake even further.

## Not Too Much Sugar
Sugars are carbohydrates that come in many forms.  Sugar is found naturally in fruits, some vegetables, milk, breads, cereals and grains, and is often added to foods during processing, preparation and when eating.  Added sugar and naturally occurring sugars are chemically identical and your body cannot distinguish between them.  Cake, cookies, candy and many soft drinks contain large amounts of added sugar that supply a large number of "nutritionally-empty calories."  Only very active people with high calorie needs can afford to consume any quantity of these sugar-laden foods.  **Sugar should be used sparingly** by people with low calorie needs and in moderation by most other healthy adults.  (Contrary to what many believe, the latest scientific evidence seems to indicate diets high in sugar do not cause diabetes.  Rather, scientific evidence indicates that adult-onset diabetes occurs most often in those who are overweight.)

## Common-Sense Nutrition
**1)  Know your daily weight maintenance caloric allowance**  (More about this later.).
**2)  Eat a variety of foods** within your caloric allowance. Consult the **Basic Food Groups** (page 59) to shape your eating patterns.  Try to

choose the proper quantity from each food group.

**3) Try not to consume foods containing partially-hydrogenated vegetable oil** because they are high in trans fats. This includes commercially prepared baked goods, snack foods, and processed foods, including most fast foods.

**4) Limit your intake of saturated fats.** Eat meat less often and fish and poultry more often, and use fat-free milk and milk products.

**5) When possible, select fresh and natural foods and whole-grain products,** and avoid chemical preservatives and additives, artificial and imitation foods, refined and processed foods, and foods that are mostly "nutritionally-empty calories."

**6) Eat nutritionally-dense foods** rather than calorie-dense foods.

**7) Take a daily multi-vitamin/mineral supplement.**

**8)** Before you buy, **read and understand the labels on food packages.**

## Eat Slowly

One final important point, try to **eat slowly**. This is especially vital if you are on a diet, trying to lose weight. If you are someone who eats fast, who finishes before everyone else at the table, you are not giving yourself a chance to feel full. While everyone else is still eating, you either sit there and pick, or you have seconds, taking in extra calories you could avoid if you would just slow down. To slow down, try eating smaller mouthfuls, try chewing your food more thoroughly, and try talking more at the table.

## Become a Calorie Expert

Today, most food packages in the United States are required to list certain nutritional information. The food labels on containers consist of several parts, including information on the front panel, and Nutrition Facts – usually on a side or rear panel.

The **Front Panel** often indicates if nutrients have been added – a case in point, "iodized salt" lets you know iodine has been added, and "enriched pasta" (or "enriched" grain of any type) means that thiamin, riboflavin, niacin, iron, and folic acid have been added. The **Nutrition Facts label** (such as that on the side of a cereal box) indicates the number of calories and nutrients in a serving. You can also use the label to compare similar foods. For instance, to determine which brand of a frozen dinner is lower in saturated fat, or which breakfast cereal contains more folic acid. Look at the "% Daily Value" column to determine if a food is high or low in a particular nutrient. The ingredient list on the Nutrition Facts label also discloses what is in the food, including any nutrients, fats, or sugars that have been added. Ingredients are in descending order by weight; i.e., the most abundant ingredient is listed first.

The Nutrition Facts label on food packages, listing nutrient content, makes it possible to calculate the number of calories in a serving if you know that there are roughly:

|  | Calories per gram | Calories per ounce |
|---|---|---|
| **Carbohydrates** | 4 | 110 |
| **Protein** | 4 | 110 |
| **Alcohol** | 7 | 200 |
| **Fat** | 9 | 260 |

**Example** Determine the calories in a cup (8 oz.) of whole milk. The label on a container of whole milk indicates that a cup has 11 grams of carbohydrate, 8 grams of protein and 9 grams of fat. The total calories in a cup of whole milk can be determined as follows:

11 gm carbs x 4 Cal per gm = 44 Cal
8 gm protein x 4 Cal per gm = 32 Cal
9 gms fat x 9 Cal per gram = 81 Cal
Total = 44+32+81 = <u>157 Calories</u>

In order to understand the calorie content of a meal, you must be able to estimate both the calorie value of foods as well as portion sizes. A sense of the **caloric value per ounce** of some <u>basic foods</u> are listed in Table 13. The extremes of the chart are represented by water the lowest, at zero Calories, and fat (lard) the highest at about 260 Calories per ounce. Sugar (a pure carbohydrate) is near the middle of the ranking at 110 Calories per ounce. Protein is also approximately 110 Calories per ounce but there is no pure protein food to rank. (Note, most of the calorie values shown in Table 13 on page 70 are the average of many varieties in a particular category.) Table 14 on page 71 is an expanded version of the Table 13 that includes the **Calories per ounce** of some commonly encountered foods.

If you appreciate that **most foods are some combination of water, carbs, protein, fat and fiber,** this can lead to a better understanding of why a particular food has the caloric value and rank shown in Table 14. For example, watermelon is almost entirely water, with some fiber (zero calories) and carbohydrate, with no protein or fat, and consequently has a very low 7 Calories per ounce value. A grape is again mostly water with some fiber and carbohydrate and according to the chart has only 19 Calories per ounce, but a raisin (a dried grape) is almost entirely carbohydrate and fiber with little water and thus has a value of 83 Calories per ounce – closer to the 110 Calories per ounce of a pure carbohydrate. When a food is not listed in the chart, common sense can often be used to estimate its caloric value; e.g., green beans are not listed, but judging from the ranking of similar foods a value of 6 or 7 Calories per ounce seems reasonable.

| Water | 0 | Pasta | 36 |
|---|---|---|---|
| Coffee or Tea | 1 | Fish | 42 |
| Vegetables | 7 | Eggs | 47 |
| Milk (fat free) | 10 | Poultry | 54 |
| Soft drink | 12 | Whiskey | 71 |
| Beer | 13 | Bread | 72 |
| Fruit | 15 | Meat | 97 |
| Milk (whole) | 18 | Cake | 100 |
| Potato | 23 | Sugar | 110 |
| Corn | 25 | Chocolate | 151 |
| Wine | 27 | Nuts | 175 |
| Rice | 33 | Vegetable oil | 253 |
| Beans | 34 | Lard | 260 |

**Table 13: Calorie Rank of Basic Foods**

Table 14 can also be thought of as a listing of the "caloric density" of foods. For instance, the table illustrates that eight ounces (half pound) of carrots contains about 80 Calories, or approximately the same number of calories as one ounce of hamburger at 82 Calories per ounce. (Note that the numbers in the table are approximate Calories per fluid or dry ounce.) Moreover, Table 14 in combination with a small weighing scale makes a very useful diet aide, allowing the calorie value of many food portions to be estimated quite accurately. It is a simple mater to weigh a piece of meat or a pancake, or a slice of apple pie, and multiply the weight in ounces by the calorie value per ounce (from Table 14) to determine the total number of calories. Often this approach results in more precise calorie values than those obtained from a common calorie table. described.

| Water | 0 | Peas | 20 | Liverwurst | 79 |
|---|---|---|---|---|---|
| Coffee or Tea | 1 | Yogurt (whole) | 21 | Hamburger | 82 |
| Vinegar | 3 | Potato (boiled) | 23 | Tuna (in oil) | 82 |
| Lettuce | 4 | Clams (raw) | 25 | Raisins | 83 |
| Celery | 5 | Banana | 25 | Bologna | 87 |
| Asparagus | 6 | Corn | 25 | Wheat Flakes | 89 |
| Tomato | 7 | Wine | 27 | Cake (average) | 100 |
| Spinach | 7 | Lobster | 27 | Sirloin Steak | 103 |
| Watermelon | 7 | Lentils | 30 | Cheese | 106 |
| Lemon | 8 | Scallops | 32 | Ham (baked) | 106 |
| Broccoli | 8 | Rice | 33 | Oatmeal | 107 |
| Mushrooms | 9 | Beans | 34 | Sugar | 110 |
| Cantaloupe | 10 | Pasta | 36 | Pretzels | 111 |
| Milk (fat free) | 10 | Tuna (in water) | 36 | Crackers | 114 |
| Carrots | 10 | Olives (black) | 37 | Doughnut | 117 |
| Strawberries | 11 | Blue Fish (baked) | 45 | Fudge | 117 |
| Green Pepper | 11 | Egg (boiled) | 47 | Chocolate | 151 |
| Peach | 11 | Turkey (light) | 50 | Potato Chips | 162 |
| Grapefruit | 11 | Ice Cream | 55 | Peanut Butter | 167 |
| Cola Drink | 12 | Sardines | 56 | Almonds | 171 |
| Beer | 13 | Turkey (dark) | 58 | Bacon | 175 |
| Yogurt (fat free) | 13 | Pancakes | 64 | Walnuts | 180 |
| Orange | 14 | Bread (wheat) | 69 | Butter | 205 |
| Apple | 16 | Whisky-86 proof | 71 | Mayonnaise | 205 |
| Milk (whole) | 18 | Apple Pie | 73 | Margarine | 206 |
| Cherries | 19 | Bread (white) | 77 | Vegetable Oil | 253 |
| Grapes | 19 | Jam/Jelly | 78 | Lard (fat) | 260 |

**Table 14: Calorie Rank of Common Foods**

# WEIGHT CONTROL

Because obesity and overweight are so common and public interest is so great, we are all continually assaulted by a blinding array of fad diets, miracle pills, health spas, exercise devices, reducing belts, and the like. Most people are left bewildered not knowing what to believe. The truth is that weight control, although a relatively complex issue, is governed by a set of logical, scientific principles, and the acceptance and understanding of these principles – augmented of course by desire and self-discipline – can lead you to sure and lasting weight control.

## Why Do we Gain (or Lose) Weight?

One of the greatest scientific achievements of the nineteenth century was the recognition and statement of the principle of conservation of energy by Julius Robert Von Mayer, in a classic paper that appeared in 1842 in Liebig's *Annalen der Chemie*. The principle is an inductive generalization based on observation of physical phenomenon and states that energy may be converted or transferred but cannot be created or destroyed. Then in 1847, a surgeon in the Prussian army, wrote a brilliant paper applying the principle to the sciences of physiology and chemistry. By the beginning of the twentieth century, scientific observations proved that the law of the conservation of energy also applied to the human metabolism.

According to the law of conservation of energy – as related to humans – the energy value of the food eaten (minus the energy lost in waste) equals the sum of the heat energy leaving the body plus the physical work done by the body. An overwhelming number of scientists today agree that weight change in human beings is linked to their energy balance (or imbalance), and that **weight change (lost or gained) in humans is governed by the law of the conservation of energy**. According to the conservation of energy principle:

**Weight Gain** occurs when your food energy intake is greater than the energy you expend. In this case your body stores the extra energy as fat.

**Weight Loss** occurs when your food energy intake is less than the energy you expend. In this case your body converts stored fat (and in some cases muscle) into energy.

Again according to the conservation of energy principle, when the energy value of the food you eat minus waste, equals the sum of the basal energy and the energy expended during physical activity, your body is in energy equilibrium. In this case, weight is neither gained nor lost. It follows then that:

**Weight Maintenance** occurs when your food energy intake equals the total energy expended in daily living.

## Weight Control Wisdom

The measure of energy, whether in the form of food, physical activity, or heat, is the kilocalorie (hereafter simply called the Calorie). As mentioned previously, weight loss occurs when you eat fewer calories than the calories you use in daily living. This difference in calories is referred to as the calorie deficit. How much weight you lose depends on the magnitude of the calorie deficit. In technical terms, **the calorie deficit, or calorie difference, is the driving force for weight change**. (Techies will appreciate that the calorie deficit which is the driving force for weight change is somewhat analogous to a voltage difference which is the driving force for the flow of electricity, and to a temperature difference which is the driving force for the flow of heat.)

As stated previously, you lose weight when your food energy intake is less than the total energy you expend. This difference in calories is referred to as the calorie deficit. How much weight you lose depends on the magnitude of your calorie deficit.

**Weight Loss**: Physiologists have long known that to lose one pound requires a deficit of approximately 3,500 Calories. Therefore, if a person's total calorie deficit over time is known, a simple metabolic calculation can be made to determine their weight loss over time.

For example, as will be evident later, a 30 year-old female office worker, 5' 4" and 175 pounds, expends about 2,500 Calories in day-to-day living. (In other words, if this woman eats about 2,500 Calories per day she will neither gain nor lose weight.) If she goes on a 1,500 Calorie per day diet, her daily deficit would be 2,500 – 1,500 = 1,000 Calories. In one week her deficit would be 1,000 Calories per day x 7 days = 7,000 Calories, and she should lose 7,000 / 3,500, or two pounds per week.

**Weight Gain**: Conversely, you gain weight when your food energy intake is more than the total energy you expend. This difference in calories is referred to as a calorie excess. How much weight you gain depends on the magnitude of your calorie excess. To gain one pound requires an excess of approximately 3,500 Calories. Therefore, if a person's total calorie excess over time is known, their weight gain over time can be computed.

For example, if the aforementioned female office worker eats 3,000 Calories per day, her daily excess would be 3,000 − 2,500 = 500 Calories. In one week her excess would be 500 Calories per day x 7 days = 3,500 Calories, and she would gain 3,500 / 3,500, or one pound per week.

This computation technique, however, is somewhat crude. Primarily because the preceding calculation does not account for a very important scientific fact which is covered in more detail in *Weight Loss for Women* or *Weight Loss for Men*, eBooks also published by NoPaperPress.com.

**Weight Fluctuation:** Your body weight rises and falls two to three pounds daily. Your weight is lowest before breakfast and highest in the evening before retiring. In addition, the quantity of water in your body also varies from day to day.

## The Weight Maintenance Program

In the following pages you will be introduced to the information you need to understand to successfully maintain your weight. You will then learn how to apply the information to establish your own personalized a weight maintenance plan, a plan that can lead to life-long weight control. Specifically you will learn:

**1)** How to select and use the Weight Maintenance Calorie Tables, to determine how many calories per day you may eat without gaining or losing a significant amount of weight.

**2)** How to analyze your eating habits to decide how you will spread your maintenance calories, first among the days of the week, and then over the meals of an individual day.

**3)** How to translate your weight maintenance calorie values into meal types and then actual food portions using a weight maintenance worksheet.

Each and every one of these points will be elaborated on later. This will be followed by time-tested weight maintenance tips and strategies that successful maintainers have been using for years.

## Activity Levels

But before you can choose a weight maintenance table, you need to estimate your activity level. To use the Activity-Level method, you must make a judgment as to how active you are. Admittedly, this is the least quantitative topic in this eBook. Nevertheless, it is the most practical, in daily living situations. A broad range of activity levels are defined in Table 15.

| Activity Level | Lifestyle | Description | Equivalent Walking Distance | Equivalent Pedometer Steps |
|---|---|---|---|---|
| 0 | Sedentary | Inactive most of day. Stands & walks very little. | Less than 1 mile | Less than 2100 |
| 1 | Relatively Inactive | Seated most of day. Stands & walks at most four hours, such as office workers etc. | 1 to 2 miles | 2100 to 4200 |
| 2 | Moderately Active | Stands as often as is seated, such as teachers, sales clerks, etc. | 3 to 5 miles | 6300 to 10,500 |
| 3 | Very Active | Stands & walks most of day, such as factory & construction workers, etc. | 6 to 8 miles | 12,600 to 16,800 |
| 4 | Extremely Active | Very hard physical work, such as lumber jacks, athletes in training, etc. | More than 8 miles | More than 16,800 |

**Table 15  Lifestyle Activity Levels**

To determine your Activity Level will, in most cases, require considerable thought on your part. Keep in mind that technology has reduced physical demands and that most people are not as active as their ancestors. As an aid, Table 15 matches the five Lifestyle Activity Levels to walking distances and an equivalent number of pedometer steps. Choose the option that best approximates the activity of your average day.

As used here, "sedentary" means only the amount of activity necessary to support independent living, and "relatively inactive" is appropriate for most office workers – who are not involved in an exercise program after work.

Note that the listed occupations are only a guide to be used to direct you to a starting point in the table. You must also factor in your after work activities to get a more complete idea of your activity level. For example, a school teacher on her feet a good part of the day would choose Activity Level 3 – moderately active. But if this teacher also works out five days a week, she could qualify for Activity Level 4 – or at the very least between Activity Level 3 and 4.

Once you settle on your Activity Level, you are ready to use the Weight Maintenance Calorie tables that follow.

## Selecting a Maintenance Table

First, you need to select the Weight Maintenance Calorie Table that's right for you. In this eBook you will find an updated set of 15 Weight Maintenance Calorie tables for men and women located in Appendices A and B. The tables are organized by gender, age, height and activity level. Men should use **Table AA** (page 87) to find the Weight Maintenance Calorie Table that's right for them, and Women should refer to **Table BB** (page 97) to determine the Weight Maintenance Calorie Table that applies to them.

## Using Weight Maintenance Tables

The use of the Weight Maintenance Calorie Tables is best illustrated by an example.

**Example**: Consider a 53-year-old, 5'-8", relatively inactive (Activity Level 1), woman who weighed 200 pounds at the start of her reducing diet. After losing 50 pounds, she weighed 150 pounds. Determine her weight maintenance calories before and after she lost weight.

From Table BB she finds that her Weight Maintenance Calorie table is **Table B.4** (page 101). From Table B.4 she finds that before she started her diet, when she weighed 200 pounds, her weight maintenance level was 2,741 Calories, meaning she must have been eating about 2,741 Calories of food per day. After her diet, the same table shows that in order to maintain her lower weight of 150 pounds she must restrict her food intake in the future to 2,297 Calories per day. On average, then, to neither gain nor lose weight at 150 pounds she must eat about 2,741 – 2,297 = 444 Calories per day less than she ate when she weighed 200 pounds.

## A Life-Long Struggle

A trim 43 year-old nutritionist laughs when people say, "Oh, you're so lucky to be naturally thin." Her reply, "Are you kidding. I workout and do you think I eat everything I want?"

Staying lean requires constant vigilance. In weight maintenance, it is the number of calories you eat over the long term that is important. As an illustration, the weight maintenance value of 2,297 Calories per day for the 53-year-old woman in the previous example amounts to about 838,000 Calories in a single year. Now realize that an annual error of only two percent of this total (that is roughly 16,800 Calories per year, or 46 Calories per day) would result in a weight gain of almost five pounds in one year, and the importance of knowing and adhering to your personal weight maintenance calorie value becomes apparent. In brief, **to control your weight it is the number of calories eaten over the long term that matters**.

Obviously, it would be impossible for the woman in the example to eat exactly 2,297 Calories day after day. Errors are inevitable and experience has shown that when people err they do so on the high side. They consume more calories than their maintenance value, rarely less. To allow for occasional overeating or days when don't have time to exercise, it is recommended that you plan to eat about seven percent below the calorie values in the weight maintenance tables. For the female in the example, that would result in about 2,140 Calories per day rather than the 2,297 Calories shown in the weight maintenance calorie table – leaving her room for an occasional calorie splurge, or a missed exercise session.

## Set Meals - Easier Calorie Control

Are you concerned about having to count calories? Whether on a reducing diet or trying to maintain your weight, allocating a specific number of calories for each meal makes it unnecessary to keep a running calorie tally for an entire day. Instead, you only need to monitor the number of calories eaten at each meal – and there are ways to keep even this to a minimum by utilizing a concept called "Set Meals" – a strategy not very different than the measured-food-to-eat systems used by diet plans such as Jenny Craig and NutriSystem. Except with the "Set Meals" system you control what you eat.

**A Set Meal is a food serving where the ingredients vary - but the**

meal is almost identical in calorie count and nutritional content day after day. **Any meal during the day that is completely under your control is a Set Meal candidate.**

For instance, suppose you prepare breakfast at home almost every day. Plan perhaps three set breakfasts. One might be based on cereal and fruit, another on eggs and toast, and so on. Variety is obtained by having more than one choice for a Set Meal, and by eating different kinds of cereal, or fruit, or egg preparations (scrambled, over easy, soft-boiled) – all within the same Set Meal. Once this is done, the number of calories in each of the Set Meal can be easily calculated. Then, try to plan set meals for lunch. The more Set Meals you have in a day, the less calorie counting. If you have set meals for both breakfast and lunch, then you only have to monitor dinner calories.

## Planning Eating Patterns

Weight maintenance begins once you are at your "best weight," or achieve a weight that feels right for you. Any motivational speech made at this point isn't going to be much help five and ten years down the road – when I trust you will still be in maintenance mode. Understand that if you really want to keep off the weight you have lost you will have to practice a good deal of self-discipline for a long time. Even the well motivated, however, need a good plan to succeed. The following approach is recommended:

**1)** Use the Weight Maintenance Calorie table that applies to you to determine your daily weight-maintenance calorie allowance.

**2)** Then decide on a weekly routine, i.e., how your calorie allowance is to be distributed among the days of the week. (Your caloric intake need not be the same every day of the week. It's your average calorie intake that counts.)

**3)** Next allocate your daily caloric allowance among the meals of the day according to your eating habits.

Obviously, a detailed meal plan for every possible calorie level cannot be included here, but given the information covered so far (particularly the healthy eating guidelines) it should be possible to plan eating patterns you can live with for any weight maintenance calorie allowance. (See the example that follows immediately). Granted this will take some work but in the long run it will be time well spent.

## Maintenance Eating Plan Example

Let's devise a weight maintenance eating plan for a 58-year-old man who, after losing 20 pounds, weighs 160 pounds. He is 5'-9" and describes his activity level as between 1 and 2. An engineering consultant, he works out of an office in his home.

First, from **Table A.8** (page 95) he finds his maintenance calorie level is between 2,389 and 2,642 Calories per day. (He decides to use the average which is approximately 2,516 Calories per day.) To determine how many calories per day he should plan to consume, he deducts a safety factor of seven percent from 2,516 to allow for occasional overeating (or under-exercising). The result is 2,340 Calories per day – the number of maintenance calories he plans to eat on most days. Then, he has to establish the meals he has control over (these will be his Set Meals), and also account for the foods he likes and dislikes. Because on most days he is home all day, he has control over every meal except dinner. (When his wife gets home from work, they prepare dinner together or sometimes go out to eat.)

For breakfast the man in the example likes cereal (with skim or soy milk) or eggs, and for lunch he prefers a tuna sandwich, soup or cereal (if he hasn't already had cereal for breakfast). He also wants to allow for a morning and afternoon snack. Now he is ready to layout his meal plan for every day of the week. The resulting maintenance eating plan is broadly outlined in Table 16 on the following page.

Next, he calculates the number of calories in the foods comprising his Set Meals, i.e., his breakfasts, lunches and snacks. The details behind Table 16 are in a spreadsheet (not shown here). In Table 16, Cereal (M) indicates a cereal with skim milk. (Be aware that four ounces of juice are included with every breakfast choice.) Worth noting is that every effort was made to balance the meals in a given day. To assure he is getting an adequate amount of nutrients every day, for dinner he always intends to have a large salad, at least two other vegetable servings, a starch (potato or brown rice), and a small serving of fish, poultry, lean meat, or a plant protein. His evening snack (dessert) frequently includes a glass of skim milk and yes a few cookies. (Nobody is perfect!)

**Overall variety is achieved by having different brands of cereal, different kinds of fruit, several types of nuts and seeds, different soup, and eggs prepared in various ways.** In addition, to introduce even

| | Mon | Tues | Weds | Thurs | Fri | Sat | Sun |
|---|---|---|---|---|---|---|---|
| **Breakfast** | Cereal (M) | Toast | Egg | Cereal (M) | Egg | Cereal (M) | Egg |
| **Snack** | Fruit | Yogurt & Fruit | Yogurt & Fruit | Fruit | Yogurt & Fruit | Fruit | Yogurt & Fruit |
| **Lunch** | Soup | Cereal (S) | Cereal (S) | Tuna | Cereal (S) | Tuna | Cereal (S) |
| **Snack** | Nuts & Seeds | Nuts & Seeds | Nuts & Seeds | Nuts & Seeds | Nuts & Seeds | Nuts & Seeds | Nuts & Seeds |
| **Calories** | 1,175 | 955 | 1,075 | 1,100 | 1,075 | 1,100 | 1,075 |

**Table 16: Maintenance Eating Plan**

more variety, every few months and in keeping with seasonal foods available, he will revisit his plan and make some adjustments to his Set Meals by adding and subtracting foods.

For dinner, his calorie allowance is his 2,340 maintenance calories minus the calories he has already eaten for breakfast, lunch and snacks. Notice that his calorie total (for breakfast, lunch and snacks) is not the same for every day of the week. This is not unexpected. Because it is unrealistic to assign a different dinner calorie target for every day of the week, he averages the daily totals for breakfast, lunch and snacks, and uses the average value to calculate his allowable calories for dinner. After a simple arithmetic calculation he finds that he is allowed 1,000 Calories for dinner. This dinner calorie total should satisfy the appetite of the man in the example and should be easy to stay within provided he eats well-balanced meals with "reasonable" portion sizes. To understand what "reasonable" portion sizes should look like for a 1,000-Calorie meal, at first he will probably have to count calories at dinner. After a few weeks of counting dinner calories, however, he should be able to judge what is and what is not an acceptable portion size for the different foods on his plate – without actually counting calories.

Using the Set Meal technique, he only has to judge or estimate his dinner calories to assure that he is close to his maintenance calories on a weekly basis. This plan should make it easier for him to control what he eats and maintain his new lower weight over the long haul. If you are not sure you can devise your own eating plan, seek the professional advice of a registered dietitian.

Finally, how should he manage the inevitable, i.e., when he has to attend a business luncheon, or an all-day business meeting, or he goes on a vacation? In other words, how should he handle those days when he just can't follow his weight maintenance eating plan? Briefly, he knows his maintenance eating pattern is approximately 400 Calories for breakfast, 500 Calories for lunch, 200 Calories for snacks, 1,000 Calories for dinner and 250 Calories for dessert. And if he has been following this pattern for some time, he should be able to recognize the kinds of food and the amounts (portion sizes) that make up the calories he is allowed at each meal. Then with the added understanding of how to estimate the calorie content of various foods, even when he eats out he should be able to order meals that approximate the calorie content of his weight maintenance eating plan. Lastly, if this approach does not work for him, he should realize that a day or two off his maintenance eating regimen is not the end of the world.

## How to Use Mini Diets

Many people go through life maintaining their weight without thinking about how much they eat or exercise. When they occasionally eat a bigger meal, they seem to automatically eat less at the next meal or they exercise more, or they do both. If for some reason they expend more energy, they instinctively eat more. These people are able to maintain an almost constant weight without any effort. For most of us, however, weight control is more difficult, and we must be vigilant. For us weight control is a relentless life-long challenge.

When on a weight-loss diet, check and record your progress by weighing yourself at the same time two or three days per week. Once you are in weight maintenance mode, i.e., you have reached your desired weight level, weigh in about once a week. Small, natural weight fluctuations can be ignored, but action is called for if you experience a "noteworthy" increase in weight. What is a noteworthy weight gain? For a 130-pound person a five-pound increase would be noteworthy; whereas for a 210-pound individual a ten-pound weight gain would be noteworthy. Both would signal a call to action. Incidentally, for most people, over a lifetime, noteworthy weight shifts are all but inevitable. Nevertheless, you should **consider a noteworthy weight change a warning that you may**

**be losing control of your weight and that you need to intervene to head off a potentially significant weight gain**.

If you need to lose five or ten pounds to get back to your maintenance weight, go on a short-term mini diet. See the **10-Day (1200 Calorie) Mini Diet** in Appendix C (page 104). It features 10 days of daily meal plans with recipes. Once back to your best weight, revisit and analyze your weight maintenance eating and exercise routines and make any adjustments needed to keep your weight on target. Furthermore, appreciate that in order to maintain a proper weight level you may have to go on a number of short-term mini diets over your lifetime to correct small weight maintenance calorie eating errors.

## Weight Maintenance Strategies

Everyone needs strategies to help stay on the right weight-maintenance track. Here are some time-tested techniques, listed in no particular order, that work. Pick and use those strategies that apply to your living style and you feel will be most helpful.

**Know your weight maintenance calorie level**: It's true that calorie counting is an imprecise art and you can't be expected to count calories every day for the rest of your life. But that said, if you are going to successfully maintain your weight over the long term it is extremely important for you to know your weight maintenance calorie level; i.e., the number of calories per day you can eat to neither gain nor lose weight.

In fact what you really must know is the amount of food your weight maintenance calorie goal represents, i.e., how much food you can eat every day. When starting, plan to eat according to that goal for two weeks, 30 days is even better. Let's call this a **training period**. During your maintenance training period, you will have to count calories, but during this time you will be developing an understanding and a recognition of the amount of food you can consume on a day-in-day-out basis to neither gain nor lose weight. After a two to four week training period, many people do a good job of sticking to their weight maintenance calorie goal – without actually counting calories.

**Use Set Meals** to make calorie control easier. Recall that a Set Meal is a food serving where the ingredients vary – but the meal is almost identical in calorie count and nutritional content day after day. Any meal during the day that is completely under your control is a Set Meal possibility. The more Set Meals you have in a day, the less calorie counting. Click here for a more complete discussion of Set Meals.

**Become a "calorie expert."** This important notion was covered in an earlier section (page 68). Reread if necessary.

**Learn to estimate portion sizes:** Another dilemma is judging portion size. It makes no sense to worry about whether to apportion 70 or 80 Calories per ounce for a cut of lean meat if you have no idea whether the portion you are planning to eat weighs four or ten ounces. You must learn to estimate portion sizes with reasonable accuracy. It's best to learn during your weight maintenance training period. Start by weighing and measuring the food you eat. After a couple of weeks, your eye should be adjusted to what four ounces of meat or six ounces of fish look like. At that point, you can then discontinue weighing.

Incidentally, judging the weight of meat or poultry is very important. As a guide, four ounces of meat or poultry is about the standard size of a slice of bread 4 x 4 x ¼ inch. (And calorie tables always refer to meat that has been cooked and trimmed of visible fat and bone.)

**Compensate to handle occasional overeating**. It's a fact of life that no matter how determined you are to abide by your daily calorie level, life has a way of interfering. In real life, you probably will not be able to eat the same number of calories day after day. Maybe it's your social life that interferes. Maybe you have to attend a wedding reception. Maybe an unexpected occasion arises where you know you're going to go over your daily calorie allowance. What should you do?

The way to handle the inevitable overeating is by compensating. You compensate by estimating how far you have strayed from your weight-loss diet and then make amends at the next opportunity (usually the next meal or two) – by eating less.

For instance, let's say you have to attend a business luncheon. Further, assume the meal has been pre-ordered so you have no choice but to eat what's served. At some point toward the end of the meal, make a mental estimate of the number of calories you have eaten. Suppose, even though you tried to be careful, your estimate is about 850 Calories. If your normal Set Lunch is 450 Calories, you know you have over done it by approximately 400 Calories. That night at dinner you decide to have water instead of wine, to forgo your evening snack and to take a half hour after-dinner walk. By doing this, before the end of the day, you will have compensated for the extra 400 Calories you ate at lunch.

**Eating at Restaurants, etc:** To reduce the number of calories you eat at a restaurant, try the following restaurant guidelines. First, for an appetizer order fruit juice or melon. For your main course order broiled fish, poultry or a lean cut of meat cooked as plainly as possible (no butter, stuffing, gravy). Order steamed vegetables and maybe a baked potato. Have your salad with the dressing on the side. Have fruit for dessert – or just coffee or tea. Finally, given the huge size of most restaurant meals, you can't go wrong if you **"eat half and take half home."**

Staying with your healthy, weight conscious eating plan when you are at home, in a restaurant, during the week, over a weekend, and even when you on vacation increases your chance of long-term weight control success.

**Out-of-control eating triggers:** Learn to recognize situations that trigger out-of-control eating. One way to identify food traps and emotionally triggered eating is to keep a journal. For as long as you find it helpful, record what you eat, how much you eat, when you eat, how you're feeling and how hungry you are. In time, you should see some patterns emerge. Once you understand these patterns and triggers, you can plan ahead and develop a strategy for how you'll handle these types of situations.

**Get a cookbook and a calorie reference:** Make sure you acquire a good low-calorie cookbook. Be sure the recipes cover breakfast, lunch and dinner, and all the recipes contain nutritional information, especially the number of calories per serving. In addition, obtain a comprehensive food calorie guide such as the excellent U.S. D. A. Home and Garden Bulletin No. 72: "Nutritive Value of Foods," which can be downloaded free.

**Keep a Food & Exercise Diary.** Behavior research has shown that people who keep a record of what they eat generally are more successful at maintaining their weight. How should you go about this? Keep a Food and Exercise Diaryl. Use a small notebook or your Smart Phone to record everything you eat and drink, when you exercise and for how long. Be honest and accurate. If your day doesn't go as expected, you can easily note any differences so that you can compensate at the next meal, or the next day.

**Prepare simple foods** cooked in an uncomplicated manner. Why? Because simple, uncomplicated meals usually contain fewer "hidden calories" than more elaborate dishes. For example, straightforward broiled fish with micro-waved vegetables makes a nutritious, quick, low-calorie dinner – with no "hidden calories." To add interest to foods

84

without adding calories, season with spices and condiments.

**Don't skip meals**. Start the day with your "Set Meal" breakfast and don't skip any meals. Why? First and most important, when you miss a meal your blood sugar falls. And it's well known that our body performs better when our blood sugar remains relatively constant. This implies eating regular small meals. In addition, some nutritionists believe that skipping meals may slow your metabolism and often cause you to overeat later in the day.

**Eat slowly**. This has been said before but it's worth repeating. If you eat fast, you are not giving yourself a chance to feel full. If you finish before everyone else at the table, while everyone else is still eating, you either sit there and pick, or you have seconds, taking in extra calories you could avoid if you would just slow down. To slow down, try eating smaller mouthfuls, try chewing your food more thoroughly, and try talking more at the table.

**Understand and use food labels**. When you shop for food read the "Nutrition Facts" label on food packages. On a per serving basis, the Nutrition Facts label lists calories, fat grams, carbohydrate grams, protein grams, fiber grams, sodium grams, sugar grams, etc. The "Ingredients" tells you what's in the package, starting with the most plentiful ingredient followed by the remaining ingredients in descending order.

**Choose a variety of healthy foods**. Make sure that you adhere to the guidelines discussed on page 57 to plan a nutritious eating plan. Use a shopping list, and don't shop when you're hungry. It's not out of the question to occasionally eat and enjoy small amounts of high-fat, high-calorie foods, but it's extremely important that day-in and day-out you routinely select foods that promote good health and weight maintenance.

**Maintain a vigorous exercise program**. Stay active! One of the most important things you can do to maintain your weight is to start and keep up a vigorous exercise program. Studies indicate it takes 30 to 60 minutes of moderately intense physical activity daily to maintain weight loss. Moderately intense physical activities include fast walking, swimming, etc.

Exactly what exercise you choose is really of secondary importance. What matters most is that whatever exercise you pick, you exercise consistently. Remember the key words: consistent, determined, steady, persistent, dogged, unswerving, gritty, single-minded. Consistent!

**Weigh yourself at least once a week**. People who weigh themselves at least once a week are more successful in keeping off the pounds by creating awareness. Monitoring your weight can tell you whether your efforts are working and can help you detect small weight gains before they become larger.

Personally, I weigh myself every morning. Sometimes I use this weight to decide how big a breakfast I can afford to eat!

**Build a support system**. Try to put together a support system, whether it's a friend, a family member, a trained professional, or a group of people who are in your situation. An understanding support system, especially when you start on maintenance, can often mean the difference between success and failure.

## Final Weight Maintenance Tip

There are undoubtedly some foods you know you shouldn't be eating on a regular basis but you just can't resist. Cake, pie, pastry, ice cream, chocolates and candy come to mind. All are high calorie, loaded with sugar and fat and with minimum nutritional value. Most successful maintainers only eat these irresistible treats on special occasions. Others only as a reward after a particularly hard exercise session – like a 10-mile hike or long distance cross-country skiing.

An excellent strategy is to not buy these treats in first place and certainly don't have them in your home. If they are not around you won't be tempted. The adage, "Out of sight out of mind" really works for many people who have maintained their weight over the long-term.

## Maintenance Gets Easier

Weight maintenance requires daily exercise, a healthy menu, a long-term commitment and constant vigilance. Good news: It gets easier over time. After a while, the maintainers just knew what worked and what didn't, and it became much easier and more satisfying to do what worked.

As a general rule of thumb, **if you can keep the weight off for one full year, so that you've gone through every birthday and every holiday, you've undoubtedly figured out how to maintain your weight and are well on your way to long-term success**. After two to five years, the odds are you will keep the weight off permanently. Achieving and staying at a healthy weight does take planning and effort, but the rewards are great.

# APPENDIX A

## Maintenance Tables for Men

This appendix contains nine Weight Maintenance Calorie Tables for Men. The tables cover men from 18 to 75 years, with heights ranging from 5' 0" to 6' 6", and activity levels from 0 to 4. Refer to the index shown in Table AA below to find the table that's right for you.

Go to page 75 to determine your Activity Level. You need this before choosing your personal Weight Maintenance Calorie table.

| Age | Height | Activity Levels | Table |
|-----|--------|-----------------|-------|
| 18-35 | 5' 0" to 5' 5" | 1 to 4 | **Page 88** |
| 18-35 | 5' 6" to 5' 11" | 1 to 4 | **Page 89** |
| 18-35 | 6' 0" to 6' 6" | 1 to 4 | **Page 90** |
| 36-55 | 5' 0" to 5' 5" | 0 to 3 | **Page 91** |
| 36-55 | 5' 6" to 5' 11" | 0 to 3 | **Page 92** |
| 36-55 | 6' 0" to 6' 6" | 0 to 3 | **Page 93** |
| 56-75 | 5' 0" to 5' 5" | 0 to 3 | **Page 94** |
| 56-75 | 5' 6" to 5' 11" | 0 to 3 | **Page 95** |
| 56-75 | 6' 0" to 6' 6" | 0 to 3 | **Page 96** |

**Table AA: Maintenance Tables for Men**

Once you have selected the Weight Maintenance Calorie table that's appropriate for you, return to the **Weight Maintenance Example** on page 76 for instruction on how to use the data in the table. The values in the tables are Maintenance Calories per day.

| Weight | Activity Level | | | | |
|--------|------|------|------|------|------|
| (lbs) | 0 | 1 | 2 | 3 | 4 |
| 100 | 1853 | 1922 | 2080 | 2327 | 2797 |
| 105 | 1904 | 1976 | 2142 | 2402 | 2895 |
| 110 | 1954 | 2030 | 2203 | 2475 | 2992 |
| 115 | 2003 | 2082 | 2264 | 2548 | 3088 |
| 120 | 2051 | 2134 | 2323 | 2620 | 3184 |
| 125 | 2099 | 2185 | 2383 | 2691 | 3279 |
| 130 | 2146 | 2236 | 2441 | 2762 | 3373 |
| 135 | 2192 | 2285 | 2499 | 2832 | 3467 |
| 140 | 2238 | 2335 | 2556 | 2902 | 3560 |
| 150 | 2328 | 2432 | 2669 | 3040 | 3745 |
| 160 | 2416 | 2527 | 2780 | 3175 | 3927 |
| 170 | 2503 | 2621 | 2890 | 3309 | 4108 |
| 180 | 2588 | 2713 | 2997 | 3442 | 4288 |
| 190 | 2672 | 2804 | 3104 | 3573 | 4466 |
| 200 | 2754 | 2893 | 3209 | 3703 | 4643 |
| 210 | 2835 | 2981 | 3313 | 3832 | 4819 |
| 220 | 2916 | 3069 | 3416 | 3960 | 4994 |
| 230 | 2995 | 3155 | 3518 | 4086 | 5167 |
| 240 | 3073 | 3240 | 3619 | 4212 | 5340 |
| 250 | 3150 | 3324 | 3719 | 4337 | 5512 |
| 260 | 3227 | 3407 | 3818 | 4460 | 5682 |

**Table A.1** Weight Maintenance Calories
Men 18 to 35, 5' 0" to 5' 5"

| Weight | Activity Level | | | | |
|--------|------|------|------|------|------|
| (lbs) | 0 | 1 | 2 | 3 | 4 |
| 120 | 2160 | 2245 | 2434 | 2731 | 3295 |
| 125 | 2210 | 2298 | 2495 | 2804 | 3392 |
| 130 | 2259 | 2350 | 2556 | 2877 | 3488 |
| 135 | 2307 | 2402 | 2615 | 2949 | 3583 |
| 140 | 2355 | 2453 | 2674 | 3020 | 3678 |
| 145 | 2402 | 2504 | 2733 | 3091 | 3773 |
| 150 | 2448 | 2554 | 2791 | 3161 | 3866 |
| 155 | 2494 | 2604 | 2848 | 3231 | 3960 |
| 160 | 2540 | 2653 | 2905 | 3301 | 4053 |
| 170 | 2630 | 2750 | 3018 | 3438 | 4237 |
| 180 | 2718 | 2845 | 3129 | 3574 | 4420 |
| 190 | 2805 | 2939 | 3239 | 3708 | 4601 |
| 200 | 2890 | 3031 | 3347 | 3841 | 4781 |
| 210 | 2974 | 3122 | 3454 | 3973 | 4960 |
| 220 | 3057 | 3212 | 3560 | 4103 | 5137 |
| 230 | 3139 | 3301 | 3664 | 4232 | 5313 |
| 240 | 3220 | 3389 | 3768 | 4361 | 5489 |
| 250 | 3300 | 3476 | 3871 | 4488 | 5663 |
| 260 | 3378 | 3562 | 3972 | 4615 | 5837 |
| 270 | 3457 | 3647 | 4073 | 4740 | 6009 |
| 280 | 3534 | 3731 | 4173 | 4865 | 6181 |

**Table A.2** Weight Maintenance Calories
Men 18 to 35, 5' 6" to 5' 11"

| Weight | Activity Level | | | | |
|--------|------|------|------|------|------|
| (lbs) | 0 | 1 | 2 | 3 | 4 |
| 140 | 2453 | 2551 | 2772 | 3118 | 3776 |
| 145 | 2502 | 2603 | 2832 | 3191 | 3872 |
| 150 | 2550 | 2655 | 2892 | 3262 | 3967 |
| 155 | 2598 | 2706 | 2951 | 3334 | 4062 |
| 160 | 2645 | 2756 | 3009 | 3404 | 4156 |
| 165 | 2691 | 2806 | 3067 | 3475 | 4250 |
| 170 | 2737 | 2856 | 3125 | 3545 | 4344 |
| 175 | 2783 | 2905 | 3182 | 3614 | 4436 |
| 180 | 2828 | 2954 | 3238 | 3683 | 4529 |
| 190 | 2917 | 3050 | 3350 | 3820 | 4713 |
| 200 | 3005 | 3145 | 3461 | 3955 | 4895 |
| 210 | 3092 | 3239 | 3570 | 4089 | 5076 |
| 220 | 3177 | 3331 | 3678 | 4222 | 5256 |
| 230 | 3261 | 3422 | 3785 | 4353 | 5434 |
| 240 | 3344 | 3512 | 3891 | 4484 | 5612 |
| 250 | 3426 | 3601 | 3996 | 4613 | 5788 |
| 260 | 3507 | 3689 | 4100 | 4742 | 5964 |
| 270 | 3587 | 3776 | 4203 | 4870 | 6139 |
| 280 | 3667 | 3863 | 4305 | 4997 | 6313 |
| 290 | 3745 | 3948 | 4406 | 5123 | 6486 |
| 300 | 3823 | 4033 | 4507 | 5248 | 6658 |

**Table A.3** Weight Maintenance Calories
Men 18 to 35, 6' 0" to 6' 6"

| Weight (lbs) | ACTIVITY LEVEL | | | |
|---|---|---|---|---|
| | 0 | 1 | 2 | 3 |
| 100 | 1771 | 1841 | 1999 | 2246 |
| 105 | 1820 | 1893 | 2059 | 2318 |
| 110 | 1868 | 1945 | 2119 | 2390 |
| 115 | 1915 | 1996 | 2177 | 2461 |
| 120 | 1962 | 2046 | 2236 | 2532 |
| 125 | 2008 | 2096 | 2293 | 2602 |
| 130 | 2054 | 2145 | 2350 | 2671 |
| 135 | 2098 | 2193 | 2406 | 2740 |
| 140 | 2143 | 2241 | 2462 | 2808 |
| 150 | 2230 | 2335 | 2572 | 2943 |
| 160 | 2316 | 2428 | 2681 | 3076 |
| 170 | 2400 | 2519 | 2788 | 3207 |
| 180 | 2483 | 2609 | 2893 | 3338 |
| 190 | 2564 | 2697 | 2997 | 3466 |
| 200 | 2644 | 2784 | 3100 | 3594 |
| 210 | 2723 | 2870 | 3202 | 3720 |
| 220 | 2801 | 2955 | 3302 | 3846 |
| 230 | 2878 | 3039 | 3402 | 3970 |
| 240 | 2954 | 3122 | 3501 | 4094 |
| 250 | 3029 | 3204 | 3599 | 4216 |
| 260 | 3103 | 3285 | 3696 | 4338 |

**Table A.4**  Weight Maintenance Calories
Men 36 to 55, 5' 0" to 5' 5"

| Weight (lbs) | ACTIVITY LEVEL | | | |
|---|---|---|---|---|
| | 0 | 1 | 2 | 3 |
| 120 | 2031 | 2115 | 2304 | 2601 |
| 125 | 2078 | 2166 | 2363 | 2672 |
| 130 | 2125 | 2216 | 2421 | 2742 |
| 135 | 2171 | 2265 | 2479 | 2812 |
| 140 | 2216 | 2314 | 2536 | 2881 |
| 145 | 2261 | 2363 | 2592 | 2950 |
| 150 | 2306 | 2411 | 2648 | 3018 |
| 155 | 2350 | 2459 | 2703 | 3086 |
| 160 | 2394 | 2506 | 2759 | 3154 |
| 170 | 2480 | 2599 | 2867 | 3287 |
| 180 | 2564 | 2690 | 2975 | 3419 |
| 190 | 2648 | 2781 | 3081 | 3550 |
| 200 | 2729 | 2869 | 3185 | 3679 |
| 210 | 2810 | 2957 | 3289 | 3808 |
| 220 | 2890 | 3044 | 3391 | 3935 |
| 230 | 2968 | 3129 | 3493 | 4061 |
| 240 | 3046 | 3214 | 3593 | 4186 |
| 250 | 3123 | 3298 | 3692 | 4310 |
| 260 | 3199 | 3381 | 3792 | 4434 |
| 270 | 3274 | 3463 | 3890 | 4557 |
| 280 | 3349 | 3545 | 3987 | 4679 |

**Table A.5** Weight Maintenance Calories
Men 36 to 55, 5' 6" to 5' 11"

| Weight (lbs) | ACTIVITY LEVEL | | | |
|---|---|---|---|---|
| | 0 | 1 | 2 | 3 |
| 140 | 2355 | 2453 | 2674 | 3020 |
| 145 | 2402 | 2504 | 2733 | 3091 |
| 150 | 2449 | 2554 | 2791 | 3161 |
| 155 | 2495 | 2604 | 2848 | 3231 |
| 160 | 2541 | 2653 | 2905 | 3301 |
| 165 | 2586 | 2701 | 2962 | 3370 |
| 170 | 2631 | 2750 | 3018 | 3438 |
| 175 | 2675 | 2797 | 3074 | 3506 |
| 180 | 2719 | 2845 | 3129 | 3574 |
| 190 | 2806 | 2939 | 3239 | 3708 |
| 200 | 2891 | 3031 | 3347 | 3841 |
| 210 | 2975 | 3122 | 3454 | 3973 |
| 220 | 3058 | 3212 | 3560 | 4103 |
| 230 | 3140 | 3301 | 3664 | 4232 |
| 240 | 3221 | 3389 | 3768 | 4361 |
| 250 | 3301 | 3476 | 3871 | 4488 |
| 260 | 3380 | 3562 | 3972 | 4615 |
| 270 | 3458 | 3647 | 4073 | 4740 |
| 280 | 3535 | 3731 | 4173 | 4865 |
| 290 | 3612 | 3815 | 4273 | 4989 |
| 300 | 3687 | 3897 | 4371 | 5112 |

**Table A.6**  Weight Maintenance Calories
Men 36 to 55, 6' 0" to 6' 6"

| Weight (lbs) | ACTIVITY LEVEL | | | |
|---|---|---|---|---|
| | 0 | 1 | 2 | 3 |
| 100 | 1682 | 1752 | 1910 | 2157 |
| 105 | 1729 | 1803 | 1969 | 228 |
| 110 | 1776 | 1853 | 2026 | 2298 |
| 115 | 1821 | 1902 | 2083 | 2368 |
| 120 | 1866 | 1950 | 2140 | 2436 |
| 125 | 1911 | 1998 | 2196 | 2504 |
| 130 | 1955 | 2046 | 2251 | 2572 |
| 135 | 1998 | 2092 | 2306 | 2639 |
| 140 | 2041 | 2139 | 2360 | 2706 |
| 150 | 2125 | 2230 | 2467 | 2838 |
| 160 | 2208 | 2320 | 2573 | 2968 |
| 170 | 2289 | 2408 | 2677 | 3097 |
| 180 | 2369 | 2495 | 2779 | 3224 |
| 190 | 2448 | 2581 | 2881 | 3350 |
| 200 | 2525 | 2665 | 2981 | 3475 |
| 210 | 2602 | 2749 | 3080 | 3599 |
| 220 | 2677 | 2831 | 3179 | 3722 |
| 230 | 2752 | 2913 | 3276 | 3844 |
| 240 | 2825 | 2993 | 3373 | 3965 |
| 250 | 2898 | 3073 | 3468 | 4086 |
| 260 | 2970 | 3152 | 3563 | 4205 |

**Table A.7**  Weight Maintenance Calories
Men 56 to 75, 5' 0" to 5' 5"

| Weight (lbs) | ACTIVITY LEVEL | | | |
|---|---|---|---|---|
| | 0 | 1 | 2 | 3 |
| 120 | 1927 | 2011 | 2201 | 2497 |
| 125 | 1973 | 2060 | 2258 | 2567 |
| 130 | 2018 | 2109 | 2314 | 2635 |
| 135 | 2062 | 2157 | 2370 | 2704 |
| 140 | 2106 | 2204 | 2425 | 2771 |
| 145 | 2150 | 2251 | 2480 | 2838 |
| 150 | 2192 | 2297 | 2534 | 2905 |
| 155 | 2235 | 2343 | 2588 | 2971 |
| 160 | 2277 | 2389 | 2642 | 3037 |
| 170 | 2360 | 2479 | 2748 | 3168 |
| 180 | 2442 | 2568 | 2852 | 3297 |
| 190 | 2522 | 2655 | 2955 | 3425 |
| 200 | 2601 | 2741 | 3057 | 3551 |
| 210 | 2679 | 2826 | 3158 | 3677 |
| 220 | 2756 | 2910 | 3258 | 3801 |
| 230 | 2832 | 2993 | 3357 | 3925 |
| 240 | 2907 | 3075 | 3455 | 4047 |
| 250 | 2982 | 3157 | 3552 | 4169 |
| 260 | 3055 | 3237 | 3648 | 4290 |
| 270 | 3128 | 3317 | 3744 | 4411 |
| 280 | 3201 | 3397 | 3839 | 4531 |

**Table A.8**  Weight Maintenance Calories
Men 56 to 75, 5' 6" to 5' 11"

| Weight (lbs) | ACTIVITY LEVEL | | | |
|---|---|---|---|---|
| | 0 | 1 | 2 | 3 |
| 140 | 2237 | 2335 | 2556 | 2902 |
| 145 | 2282 | 2384 | 2613 | 2971 |
| 150 | 2327 | 2432 | 2669 | 3040 |
| 155 | 2371 | 2480 | 2725 | 3108 |
| 160 | 2415 | 2527 | 2780 | 3175 |
| 165 | 2459 | 2574 | 2835 | 3243 |
| 170 | 2502 | 2621 | 2890 | 3309 |
| 175 | 2545 | 2667 | 2944 | 3376 |
| 180 | 2587 | 2713 | 2997 | 3442 |
| 190 | 2671 | 2804 | 3104 | 3573 |
| 200 | 2753 | 2893 | 3209 | 3703 |
| 210 | 2834 | 2981 | 3313 | 3832 |
| 220 | 2915 | 3069 | 3416 | 3960 |
| 230 | 2994 | 3155 | 3518 | 4086 |
| 240 | 3072 | 3240 | 3619 | 4212 |
| 250 | 3149 | 3324 | 3719 | 4337 |
| 260 | 3225 | 3407 | 3817 | 4460 |
| 270 | 3301 | 3490 | 3917 | 4584 |
| 280 | 3376 | 3572 | 4014 | 4706 |
| 290 | 3450 | 3653 | 4111 | 4828 |
| 300 | 3524 | 3734 | 4208 | 4949 |

**Table A.9** Weight Maintenance Calories
Men 56 to 75, 6' 0" to 6' 6"

# APPENDIX B

## Maintenance Tables for Women

This appendix contains six Weight Maintenance Calorie Tables for Women. The tables cover women from 18 to 75 years, with heights ranging from 4' 11" to 6' 0", and activity levels from 0 to 4. Refer to the index shown in Table BB below to find the table that's right for you. In addition, go to page 75 to determine your Activity Level. You need this before choosing your personal Weight Maintenance Calorie table.

| Age | Height | Activity Levels | Table |
|---|---|---|---|
| 18 - 35 | 4' 11" to 5' 5" | 1 to 4 | **Page 98** |
| 18 - 35 | 5' 6" to 6' 0" | 1 to 4 | **Page 99** |
| 36 - 55 | 4' 11" to 5' 5" | 0 to 3 | **Page 100** |
| 36 - 55 | 5' 6" to 6' 0" | 0 to 3 | **Page 101** |
| 56 - 75 | 4' 11" to 5' 5" | 0 to 3 | **Page 102** |
| 56 - 75 | 5' 6" to 6' 0" | 0 to 3 | **Page 103** |

**Table BB: Maintenance Tables for Women**

Once you have selected the Weight Maintenance Calorie table that's appropriate for you, go to the **Weight Maintenance Example** (page 76) to see how to use the table. Recall the values in the tables are Maintenance Calories per day.

| Weight | Activity Level | | | | |
|---|---|---|---|---|---|
| (lbs) | 0 | 1 | 2 | 3 | 4 |
| 100 | 1729 | 1799 | 1956 | 2204 | 2677 |
| 105 | 1777 | 1851 | 2016 | 2276 | 2772 |
| 110 | 1824 | 1901 | 2074 | 2347 | 2867 |
| 115 | 1870 | 1951 | 2132 | 2417 | 2961 |
| 120 | 1916 | 2001 | 2190 | 2487 | 3054 |
| 125 | 1962 | 2050 | 2246 | 2556 | 3147 |
| 130 | 2006 | 2098 | 2302 | 2624 | 3239 |
| 135 | 2050 | 2145 | 2358 | 2692 | 3331 |
| 140 | 2094 | 2193 | 2413 | 2759 | 3422 |
| 145 | 2137 | 2239 | 2467 | 2826 | 3512 |
| 150 | 2180 | 2286 | 2522 | 2893 | 3602 |
| 160 | 2264 | 2377 | 2629 | 3025 | 3781 |
| 170 | 2347 | 2467 | 2734 | 3155 | 3959 |
| 180 | 2428 | 2555 | 2838 | 3284 | 4135 |
| 190 | 2508 | 2642 | 2941 | 3411 | 4310 |
| 200 | 2587 | 2728 | 3042 | 3537 | 4483 |
| 210 | 2665 | 2813 | 3143 | 3663 | 4656 |
| 220 | 2741 | 2896 | 3242 | 3787 | 4827 |
| 230 | 2817 | 2979 | 3341 | 3910 | 4998 |
| 240 | 2892 | 3061 | 3439 | 4033 | 5168 |
| 250 | 2966 | 3142 | 3535 | 4154 | 5337 |

**Table B.1**  Weight Maintenance Calories
Women 18 to 35, 4' 11" to 5' 5"

| Weight | Activity Level | | | | |
|---|---|---|---|---|---|
| (lbs) | 0 | 1 | 2 | 3 | 4 |
| 100 | 1820 | 1890 | 2048 | 2295 | 2770 |
| 105 | 1870 | 1944 | 2110 | 2369 | 2868 |
| 110 | 1919 | 1996 | 2170 | 2442 | 2964 |
| 115 | 1968 | 2048 | 2230 | 2514 | 3060 |
| 120 | 2015 | 2099 | 2289 | 2585 | 3155 |
| 125 | 2062 | 2150 | 2347 | 2656 | 3250 |
| 130 | 2109 | 2200 | 2405 | 2726 | 3343 |
| 135 | 2155 | 2249 | 2463 | 2796 | 3437 |
| 140 | 2200 | 2298 | 2519 | 2865 | 3529 |
| 145 | 2245 | 2346 | 2575 | 2934 | 3622 |
| 150 | 2289 | 2394 | 2631 | 3002 | 3713 |
| 160 | 2376 | 2488 | 2741 | 3136 | 3895 |
| 170 | 2462 | 2581 | 2850 | 3270 | 4076 |
| 180 | 2546 | 2672 | 2957 | 3401 | 4255 |
| 190 | 2629 | 2762 | 3062 | 3531 | 4433 |
| 200 | 2710 | 2850 | 3166 | 3660 | 4609 |
| 210 | 2791 | 2938 | 3270 | 3788 | 4784 |
| 220 | 2870 | 3024 | 3372 | 3915 | 4958 |
| 230 | 2948 | 3109 | 3473 | 4041 | 5131 |
| 240 | 3026 | 3194 | 3573 | 4166 | 5303 |
| 250 | 3102 | 3277 | 3672 | 4290 | 5475 |

**Table B.2**  Weight Maintenance Calories
Women 18 to 35 yrs, 5' 6" to 6' 0"

| Weight | ACTIVITY LEVEL | | | |
|---|---|---|---|---|
| (lbs) | 0 | 1 | 2 | 3 |
| 100 | 1682 | 1752 | 1910 | 2157 |
| 105 | 1729 | 1803 | 1969 | 2228 |
| 110 | 1776 | 1853 | 2026 | 2298 |
| 115 | 1821 | 1902 | 2083 | 2368 |
| 120 | 1866 | 1950 | 2140 | 2436 |
| 125 | 1911 | 1998 | 2196 | 2504 |
| 130 | 1955 | 2046 | 2251 | 2572 |
| 135 | 1998 | 2092 | 2306 | 2639 |
| 140 | 2041 | 2139 | 2360 | 2706 |
| 145 | 2083 | 2185 | 2414 | 2772 |
| 150 | 2125 | 2230 | 2467 | 2838 |
| 160 | 2208 | 2320 | 2573 | 2968 |
| 170 | 2289 | 2408 | 2677 | 3097 |
| 180 | 2369 | 2495 | 2779 | 3224 |
| 190 | 2448 | 2581 | 2881 | 3350 |
| 200 | 2525 | 2665 | 2981 | 3475 |
| 210 | 2602 | 2749 | 3080 | 3599 |
| 220 | 2677 | 2831 | 3179 | 3722 |
| 230 | 2752 | 2913 | 3276 | 3844 |
| 240 | 2825 | 2993 | 3373 | 3965 |
| 250 | 2898 | 3073 | 3468 | 4086 |

**Table B.3** Weight Maintenance Calories
Women 36 to 55, 4' 11" to 5' 5"

| Weight (lbs) | ACTIVITY LEVEL | | | |
|---|---|---|---|---|
| | 0 | 1 | 2 | 3 |
| 100 | 1739 | 1809 | 1967 | 2214 |
| 105 | 1787 | 1861 | 2027 | 2286 |
| 110 | 1835 | 1912 | 2085 | 2357 |
| 115 | 1881 | 1962 | 2144 | 2428 |
| 120 | 1927 | 2011 | 2201 | 2497 |
| 125 | 1973 | 2060 | 2258 | 2567 |
| 130 | 2018 | 2109 | 2314 | 2635 |
| 135 | 2062 | 2157 | 2370 | 2704 |
| 140 | 2106 | 2204 | 2425 | 2771 |
| 145 | 2150 | 2251 | 2480 | 2838 |
| 150 | 2192 | 2297 | 2534 | 2905 |
| 160 | 2277 | 2389 | 2642 | 3037 |
| 170 | 2360 | 2479 | 2748 | 3168 |
| 180 | 2442 | 2568 | 2852 | 3297 |
| 190 | 2522 | 2655 | 2955 | 3425 |
| 200 | 2601 | 2741 | 3057 | 3551 |
| 210 | 2679 | 2826 | 3158 | 3677 |
| 220 | 2756 | 2910 | 3258 | 3801 |
| 230 | 2832 | 2993 | 3357 | 3925 |
| 240 | 2907 | 3075 | 3455 | 4047 |
| 250 | 2982 | 3157 | 3552 | 4169 |

**Table B.4** Weight Maintenance Calories
Women 36 to 55, 5' 6" to 6' 0"

| Weight (lbs) | ACTIVITY LEVEL | | | |
|---|---|---|---|---|
| | 0 | 1 | 2 | 3 |
| 100 | 1608 | 1678 | 1836 | 2083 |
| 105 | 1653 | 1727 | 1893 | 2152 |
| 110 | 1698 | 1775 | 1949 | 2221 |
| 115 | 1742 | 1823 | 2005 | 2289 |
| 120 | 1786 | 1870 | 2060 | 2356 |
| 125 | 1829 | 1916 | 2114 | 2423 |
| 130 | 1871 | 1962 | 2168 | 2489 |
| 135 | 1913 | 2008 | 2221 | 2555 |
| 140 | 1955 | 2053 | 2274 | 2620 |
| 145 | 1996 | 2098 | 2327 | 2685 |
| 150 | 2037 | 2142 | 2379 | 2749 |
| 160 | 2117 | 2229 | 2482 | 2877 |
| 170 | 2196 | 2315 | 2584 | 3003 |
| 180 | 2274 | 2400 | 2684 | 3129 |
| 190 | 2350 | 2483 | 2783 | 3252 |
| 200 | 2425 | 2565 | 2881 | 3375 |
| 210 | 2500 | 2647 | 2978 | 3497 |
| 220 | 2573 | 2727 | 3075 | 3618 |
| 230 | 2646 | 2807 | 3170 | 3738 |
| 240 | 2717 | 2885 | 3265 | 3857 |
| 250 | 2789 | 2964 | 3359 | 3976 |

**Table B.5**  Weight Maintenance Calories
Women 56 to 75, 4' 11" to 5' 5"

| Weight | ACTIVITY LEVEL | | | |
|:---:|:---:|:---:|:---:|:---:|
| (lbs) | 0 | 1 | 2 | 3 |
| 100 | 1665 | 1735 | 1893 | 2140 |
| 105 | 1711 | 1785 | 1951 | 2210 |
| 110 | 1757 | 1834 | 2008 | 2280 |
| 115 | 1803 | 1883 | 2065 | 2349 |
| 120 | 1847 | 1931 | 2121 | 2417 |
| 125 | 1891 | 1979 | 2176 | 2485 |
| 130 | 1935 | 2026 | 2231 | 2552 |
| 135 | 1978 | 2072 | 2286 | 2619 |
| 140 | 2020 | 2118 | 2340 | 2685 |
| 145 | 2062 | 2164 | 2393 | 2751 |
| 150 | 2104 | 2209 | 2446 | 2817 |
| 160 | 2186 | 2298 | 2551 | 2946 |
| 170 | 2267 | 2386 | 2655 | 3074 |
| 180 | 2346 | 2472 | 2757 | 3201 |
| 190 | 2424 | 2557 | 2858 | 3327 |
| 200 | 2501 | 2641 | 2957 | 3451 |
| 210 | 2577 | 2724 | 3056 | 3575 |
| 220 | 2652 | 2806 | 3154 | 3697 |
| 230 | 2726 | 2887 | 3251 | 3819 |
| 240 | 2800 | 2968 | 3347 | 3940 |
| 250 | 2872 | 3047 | 3442 | 4060 |

**Table B.6**  Weight Maintenance Calories
Women 56 to 75, 5' 6" to 6' 0"

# <u>APPENDIX C</u>

## 10-Day Mini Diet

Use the following short-term mini diet if you need to lose five or ten pounds to get back to your maintenance weight.

## 1200 Calorie Meal Plans

The following mini diet has 1,200 Calories per day. If 1,200 Calories is too drastic for you, add some of these snacks to increase the calorie total: Handful of unsalted mixed nuts (100 Calories), Medium size banana (100 Calories), Fresh fruit in season - apple, pear, peach, etc (70 Calories), Yogurt 6 oz – nonfat (90 Calories), Skinny Cow Ice Cream Sandwich (140 Calories), and Kashi TLC Chewy Granola Bar (140 Calories).

The recipes associated with the meal plans are courtesy of Gail Johnson and NoPaperPress.com.

# Day 1 – 1200 Calorie Meal Plan

| BREAKFAST | Calories | Totals |
|---|---|---|
| Orange juice (½ cup) | 50 | |
| Wheaties (¾ cup) + ½ cup skim milk + ½ banana | 190 | |
| Coffee | 10 | 250 Cal |
| | | |
| **SNACK** | | |
| Fresh fruit in season (apple, pear, peach, etc) | 70 | |
| Coffee or tea | 10 | 80 Cal |
| | | |
| **LUNCH** | | |
| Vegetable soup (1 cup) | 110 | |
| Turkey breast (1 oz) on 1 slice rye bread (½ | 105 | |
| Lettuce & tomato slices | 20 | |
| Skim milk (4 ounces) | 40 | 275 Cal |
| | | |
| **SNACK** | | |
| One small chocolate chip cookie | 80 | |
| Coffee or tea | 10 | 90 Cal |
| | | |
| **DINNER** | | |
| Baked Herb-Crusted Cod (Day 1 Recipe - page 115) | 230 | |
| Spinach (½ cup) steamed w garlic & drizzled w Evoo | 100 | |
| Asparagus (7 spears cooked & drained) | 20 | |
| Whole grain bread (1 slice) | 65 | |
| Water | 0 | 415 Cal |
| | | |
| **SNACK** | | |
| Popcorn (5 cups plain hot-air popped) | 80 | |
| Coffee or tea | 10 | 90 Cal |
| | | |
| | | 1200 Cal |

# Day 2 – 1200 Calorie Meal Plan

| BREAKFAST | Calories | Totals |
|---|---|---|
| Fresh or frozen strawberries (½ cup) | 25 | |
| French toasted English Muffin (Day 2 Recipe - page 116) | 270 | |
| Light syrup (1 Tbsp) | 30 | |
| Coffee | 10 | 335 Cal |
| | | |
| **SNACK** | | |
| Coffee or tea | 10 | 10 Cal |
| | | |
| **LUNCH** | | |
| Salad (3 oz tuna, 1 tsp Evoo, onions & celery) | 175 | |
| Lettuce & tomato wedges | 20 | |
| Fresh fruit in season (apple, pear, peach, etc) | 70 | |
| Coffee or tea | 10 | 275 Cal |
| | | |
| **SNACK** | | |
| Yogurt (6 oz – nonfat, any flavor) | 90 | |
| Coffee or tea | 10 | 100 Cal |
| | | |
| **DINNER** | | |
| Broiled veal chop (4 oz lean) | 200 | |
| Corn on the cob (1 medium ear) | 100 | |
| Broccoli (½ cup steamed) | 25 | |
| Large green salad with 1½ Tbsp low-cal dressing | 70 | |
| Water | 0 | 395 Cal |
| | | |
| **SNACK** | | |
| Graham crackers (3 squares) | 90 | |
| Coffee or tea | 10 | 100 Cal |
| | | |
| | | 1215 Cal |

# Day 3 – 1200 Calorie Meal Plan

| BREAKFAST | Calories | Totals |
|---|---|---|
| Grapefruit (½) | 75 | |
| Scrambled egg | 80 | |
| Whole wheat toast (1 slice) | 65 | |
| Coffee | 10 | 230 Cal |
| | | |
| **SNACK** | | |
| Coffee or tea | 10 | 10 Cal |
| | | |
| **LUNCH** | | |
| Ham sandwich (2 oz ham & 1 slice rye bread) | 225 | |
| Small bunch of grapes | 65 | |
| Hot or iced tea | 10 | 300 Cal |
| | | |
| **SNACK** | | |
| Fresh fruit in season (apple, peach, plum, etc) | 70 | |
| Coffee or tea | 10 | 80 Cal |
| | | |
| **DINNER** | | |
| Chicken w Peppers & Onions (Day 3 Recipe - page 117) | 250 | |
| Sautéed red peppers with onions | 70 | |
| Green beans - steamed & mashed cauliflower | 55 | |
| Large green salad with 1½ Tbsp low-cal dressing | 70 | |
| Skim milk (4 oz) | 40 | 485 Cal |
| | | |
| **SNACK** | | |
| Popcorn (5 cups plain hot-air popped) | 80 | |
| Coffee or tea | 10 | 90 Cal |
| | | |
| | | 1195 Cal |

# Day 4 – 1200 Calorie Meal Plan

| BREAKFAST | Calories | Totals |
|---|---|---|
| Grapefruit (½) | 75 | |
| Cheerios (1 cup) + ½ cup skim milk + 15 raisins | 190 | |
| Coffee | 10 | 275 Cal |
| | | |
| **SNACK** | | |
| Coffee or tea | 10 | 10 Cal |
| | | |
| **LUNCH** | | |
| Cottage cheese (1 cup low fat) | 180 | |
| Large green salad 1½ Tbsp low-cal dressing | 70 | |
| Small whole-grain roll | 80 | |
| Hot or iced tea | 10 | 340 Cal |
| | | |
| **SNACK** | | |
| Fresh fruit in season (apple, peach, plum, etc) | 70 | |
| Coffee or tea | 10 | 80 Cal |
| | | |
| **DINNER** | | |
| Meat Loaf (Day 4 Recipe - page 118) | 290 | |
| One-half acorn squash (½ tsp maple syrup) | 90 | |
| Spinach (½ cup steamed & drizzled 1 tsp Evoo) | 70 | |
| Romaine lettuce, tomato slice, 1 Tbsp low-cal | 45 | |
| Water | 0 | 495 Cal |
| | | |
| **SNACK** | | |
| Coffee or tea | 10 | 10 Cal |
| | | |
| | | 1210 Cal |

# Day 5 – 1200 Calorie Meal Plan

| BREAKFAST | Calories | Totals |
|---|---|---|
| Cantaloupe (½ medium) | 50 | |
| Fried egg | 80 | |
| Toasted raisin bread (1 slice) | 75 | |
| Coffee | 10 | 215 Cal |
| | | |
| **SNACK** | | |
| Coffee or tea | 10 | 10 Cal |
| | | |
| **LUNCH** | | |
| Beef barley soup (1 cup) | 145 | |
| Small whole-grain roll | 80 | |
| Lettuce, sliced tomato 1 Tbsp low-cal dressing | 45 | |
| Canned pineapple (½ cup, no-sugar-added juice) | 40 | |
| Hot or iced tea | 10 | 320 Cal |
| | | |
| **SNACK** | | |
| Yogurt (6 oz nonfat, any flavor) | 90 | |
| Coffee or tea | 10 | 100 Cal |
| | | |
| **DINNER** | | |
| Frozen fish dinner (Day 5 Recipe - page 119) | 340 | |
| Large green salad 1½ Tbsp low-cal dressing | 70 | |
| Skim milk (6oz) | 60 | |
| Fresh fruit in season (apple, peach, plum, etc) | 70 | |
| Water | 0 | 540 Cal |
| | | |
| **SNACK** | | |
| Coffee or tea | 10 | 10 Cal |
| | | |
| | | 1195 Cal |

# Day 6 – 1200 Calorie Meal Plan

| BREAKFAST | Calories | Totals |
|---|---|---|
| Tomato juice (½ cup) | 20 | |
| **Shredded Wheat** (1 cup) + ½ cup skim milk + ½ | 265 | |
| Coffee | 10 | 295 Cal |
| | | |
| **SNACK** | | |
| Coffee or tea | 10 | 10 Cal |
| | | |
| **LUNCH** | | |
| Leftover meat loaf  (½ Day 4 serving size) | 155 | |
| Small whole-grain roll | 80 | |
| Lettuce | 0 | |
| Fresh or frozen berries (½ cup) | 50 | |
| Hot or iced tea | 10 | 295 Cal |
| | | |
| **SNACK** | | |
| Yogurt (6 oz  nonfat, any flavor) | 90 | |
| Coffee or tea | 10 | 100 Cal |
| | | |
| **DINNER** | | |
| Pizza (**Day 6 Recipe** - page 120) | 350 | |
| Large green salad 1½ Tbsp low-cal dressing | 70 | |
| Fresh fruit in season (apple, peach, plum, etc) | 70 | |
| Water | 0 | 490 Cal |
| | | |
| **SNACK** | | |
| Coffee or tea | 10 | 10 Cal |
| | | |
| | | 1200 Cal |

# Day 7 – 1200 Calorie Meal Plan

| BREAKFAST | Calories | Totals |
|---|---|---|
| Cantaloupe (½ medium) | 50 | |
| Oatmeal (½ cup dry) + ½ cup skim milk + 15 | 220 | |
| Coffee | 10 | 280 Cal |
| | | |
| **SNACK** | | |
| Coffee or tea | 10 | 10 Cal |
| | | |
| **LUNCH** | | |
| Grilled cheese sandwich (2 slices 2% cheese) | 230 | |
| Lettuce and sliced tomato | 20 | |
| Pickle spears | 0 | |
| Water | 0 | 250 Cal |
| | | |
| **SNACK** | | |
| Carrot sticks with ¼ cup low-fat cottage cheese & | 60 | |
| Coffee or tea | 10 | 70 Cal |
| | | |
| **DINNER** | | |
| Eat Out – Chicken dinner Day 7 Recipe - page 121 | | |
| Max allowable calories | 580 | |
| Water | 0 | 580 Cal |
| | | |
| **SNACK** | | |
| Coffee or tea | 10 | 10 Cal |
| | | |
| | | 1200 Cal |

# Day 8 – 1200 Calorie Meal Plan

| BREAKFAST | Calories | Totals |
|---|---|---|
| Cantaloupe (½ medium) | 50 | |
| Wheaties (¾ cup) + ½ cup skim milk + ½ banana | 190 | |
| Coffee | 10 | 250 Cal |
| | | |
| **SNACK** | | |
| Coffee or tea | 10 | 10 Cal |
| | | |
| **LUNCH** | | |
| Lentil soup (1 cup) | 140 | |
| Turkey (1 oz) on 1 slice of rye bread | 115 | |
| Lettuce & tomato slices | 20 | |
| Skim milk (4 oz) | 40 | 315 Cal |
| | | |
| **SNACK** | | |
| Coffee or tea | 10 | 10 Cal |
| | | |
| **DINNER** | | |
| Baked salmon w salsa Day 8 Recipe - page 122 | 215 | |
| Summer squash, zucchini and tomatoes | 60 | |
| Brown rice (½ cup) | 100 | |
| Large green salad with 1½ Tbsp low-cal dressing | 70 | |
| Fresh fruit in season (apple, peach, plum, etc) | 70 | |
| Water | 0 | 515 Cal |
| | | |
| **SNACK** | | |
| Popcorn (6 cups plain hot-air popped) | 100 | |
| Coffee or tea | 10 | 110 Cal |
| | | |
| | | 1210 Cal |

# Day 9 – 1200 Calorie Meal Plan

| BREAKFAST | Calories | Totals |
|---|---|---|
| Orange juice (½ cup) | 50 | |
| Soft-boiled egg + whole wheat toast (1 slice) | 145 | |
| Coffee | 10 | 205 Cal |
| | | |
| **SNACK** | | |
| Coffee or tea | 10 | 10 Cal |
| | | |
| **LUNCH** | | |
| Salad (3 oz tuna, 1 tsp Evoo, onions & celery) | 175 | |
| Lettuce & tomato wedges | 20 | |
| Rye bread ( 1 slice) | 65 | |
| Fresh fruit in season – (apple, pear, peach, etc) | 70 | |
| Coffee or tea | 10 | 340 Cal |
| | | |
| **SNACK** | | |
| Yogurt (6 oz  nonfat, any flavor) | 90 | |
| Coffee or tea | 10 | 100 Cal |
| | | |
| **DINNER** | | |
| Veggie burger (1 patty) (Day 9 Recipe - page 123) | 100 | |
| Low-fat cheddar cheese (1 thin slice) +  3 Beets | 50 | |
| Seeded hamburger roll | 140 | |
| Large green salad 1½ Tbsp low-cal dressing | 70 | |
| Fresh fruit in season (apple, peach, plum, etc) | 70 | |
| Skim milk (6 oz) | 60 | 535 Cal |
| | | |
| **SNACK** | | |
| Coffee or tea | 10 | 10 Cal |
| | | |
| | | 1200 Cal |

# Day 10 – 1200 Calorie Meal Plan

| BREAKFAST | Calories | Totals |
|---|---|---|
| Orange juice (½ cup) | 50 | |
| Wild blueberry pancakes Day 10 Recipe - page 124 | 190 | |
| Light syrup (1 Tbsp) | 30 | |
| Coffee | 10 | 280 Cal |
| | | |
| **SNACK** | | |
| Coffee or tea | 10 | 10 Cal |
| | | |
| **LUNCH** | | |
| Peanut butter (2 Tbsp) on 2 slices of whole-grain | 330 | |
| Skim milk (8 ounces) | 90 | |
| Fresh fruit in season (apple, peach, plum, etc) | 70 | 490 Cal |
| | | |
| **SNACK** | | |
| Coffee or tea | 10 | 10 Cal |
| | | |
| **DINNER** | | |
| Vegetable bouillon | 0 | |
| Broiled pork chop (about ½" thick, trimmed of fat) | 260 | |
| Green peas (½ cup) | 55 | |
| Tomato & cucumber salad with 2 Tbsp low-cal | 70 | |
| Water with lemon section | 15 | 400 Cal |
| | | |
| **SNACK** | | |
| Coffee or tea | 10 | 10 Cal |
| | | |
| | | 1200 Cal |

# Recipes for Mini Diet

## Day 1 - Recipe

### Baked Cod

    4  cod fish fillets (4 to 5 ounces each)
    2  tablespoons flour
    2  tablespoons cornmeal
    2  tablespoons minced fresh herbs
    2  teaspoons lemon juice

Sprinkle cod with lemon juice. Mix flour, cornmeal and herbs and dust the cod with the cornmeal-herb mixture.  Bake in oven at 375 °F for 10 minutes.  Add salt and black pepper to taste.

**Serves 4**.  One serving is 230 Calories (cod only).

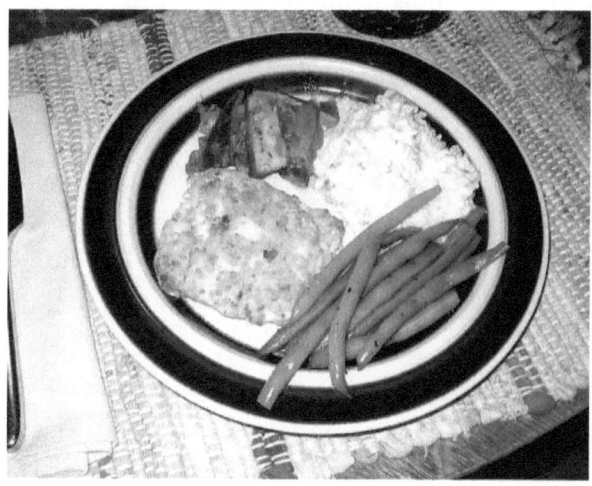

# Day 2 - Recipe
## French-Toasted English Muffin

    6 whole wheat English muffins (light)
    4 eggs
    2 cups skim milk
    2 teaspoons (tsp) vanilla
    Dash of cinnamon

In a medium bowl, beat together eggs and skim milk. Add vanilla and cinnamon. Separate English muffins into halves and saturate slices in egg mixture. In a non-stick skillet coated with cooking spray, cook muffins until both sides are golden brown. Dust lightly with confectionary sugar. Serve hot or keep in an oven or warmer at 200 °F until ready to plate.
**Serves 4**. Three English muffin slices (1½ muffins) per serving. Serving is 270 Calories.

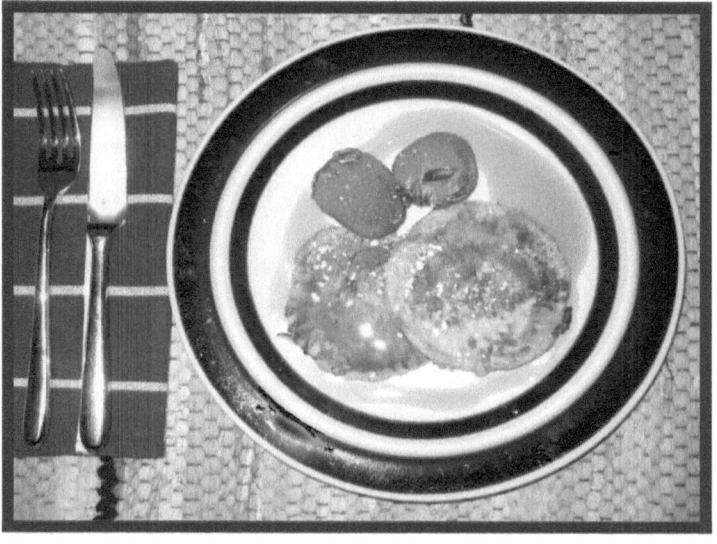

# Day 3- Recipe
## Chicken with Peppers & Onions

4 boneless & skinless chicken breasts (~ 5 oz each)

Coat the chicken breasts in a bottled barbeque sauce. Prepare medium-hot fire on well-oiled gas or charcoal grill . Place breasts on grill, turning them every 4 minutes, for 10 to 12 minutes, or until done. (To check if breasts are done, the meat should be moist and white with no sign of pink when you cut into breast.) Serve hot.

2 medium red peppers

1 medium onion

Place peppers and onions in pan with 2 Tbsp fat-free chicken stock. Sauté until stock is reduced. Spray pan lightly with non-stick cooking oil and sauté another 2 minutes. Salt and pepper to taste.

**Serves 4**. About 250 Calories per serving (for chicken only).

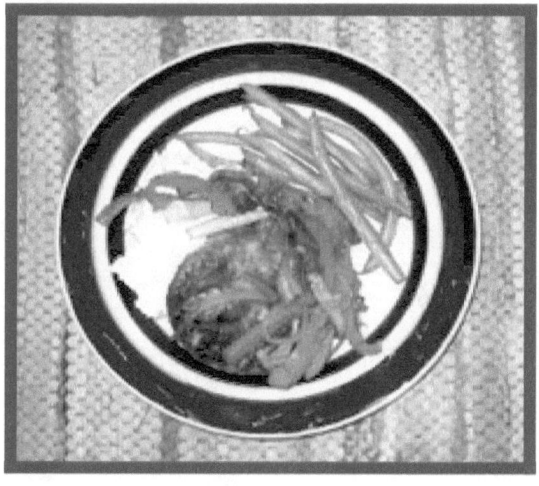

# Day 4 - Recipe

## Meat Loaf

½ pound ground white meat turkey
½ pound ground beef (about 90% lean)
1 large egg
½ cup skim milk
¼ cup bread crumbs
¼ cup ketchup
¼ cup chopped carrots
¼ cup chopped onion

In a medium bowl, combine all ingredients. Add salt and pepper to taste.
Mix until blended and form into a loaf. Place loaf into oven preheated to
350 °F. Bake until an instant-read thermometer inserted in the center of
the loaf reads 160 °F. This should take about one hour.

Shown below is meat loaf, acorn squash baked with 1 tsp maple syrup and
steamed spinach drizzled with extra-virgin olive oil (Evoo).

**Serves 5**. Each serving of meat loaf is about 290 Calories (for meat loaf
only).

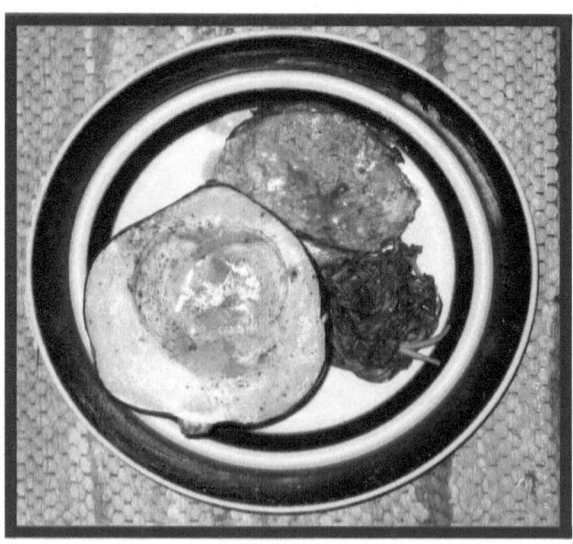

# Day 5 - Recipe

## Frozen-Fish Dinner

No recipe today.  No cooking today.  It's your day off!  Some reasonably good frozen fish dinners are:

- Lean Cuisine Shrimp Alfredo (160 Cal)
- Smart Ones Tuna Noodle Casserole (250 Cal)
- Lean Cuisine Tortilla Crusted Fish (300 Cal)

That's it.  There are just not that many frozen fish dinners for sale at supermarkets.  If you choose "Salmon with Lemon Dill Sauce" or "Shrimp with Vegetables," you will not use all of the **340 Calories allocated for this Day 5 meal**.  In this case, use the excess 100 or so calories anyway you wish.  Splurge on extra dessert or save the calories for the next day and have a larger piece of pizza!

# Day 6 - Recipe

## Grandma's Pizza

The following is a pizza recipe used by my Italian grandmother. She was from a small mountain village located between Rome and Naples.

**Pizza dough:** To save time use prepared dough, preferably whole wheat. Flour a large cutting board. <u>Divide one pound of prepared pizza dough into four parts.</u> Roll out each dough ball as thin as possible.

**Tomato sauce:** Sauté ½ small onion, chopped fine, in 1 tsp olive oil. Add two finely chopped garlic cloves, 1½ cups chopped plum tomatoes and ½ tsp chopped fresh oregano. Stir and cook about 5 minutes on a low flame.

**Pizza preparation & cooking:** On each pizza, spread evenly about ¼ cup of the tomato sauce. Add about ½ ounce of shredded part-skim mozzarella cheese, 1 tsp Parmesan cheese, 3 slices of a Portobello mushroom, some torn fresh basil, and drizzle with Evoo. Put pizzas on a pan and place in 475 °F oven for about 15 to 20 minutes, or until crust is crisp and cheese is just melting. (Freeze left over sauce for a future meal..)

<u>Serves 4</u>. Make four pizzas. Each pizza contains about 350 Calories.

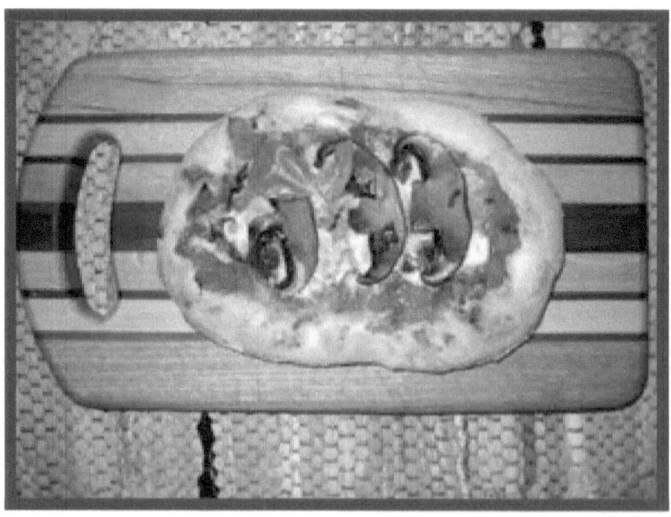

# Day 7 - Recipe

## Chicken Dinner - Out

No recipe today. No cooking today. Have a chicken dinner at your favorite restaurant, but make sure you choose a restaurant where you have a fighting chance to achieve your calorie goal. Your goal for dinner is a **maximum of 630 Calories**. This includes appetizer, soup, main course and dessert.

**Tips for Eating Out:** First, order simple, such as broiled chicken breast with steamed vegetables and brown rice. Tell the waiter you want no sauce, no gravy, nothing added. Then, knowing your calorie objective, and that chicken is about 50 Calories per ounce, most steamed vegetable servings average approximately 50 Calories per cup, and rice is about 100 Calories per ½ cup, decide how much to eat – and take the remainder home. If fresh fruit is not an option, pass on dessert and have the evening snack specified for that day in the diet.

In a restaurant, some nutritionists recommend you eat the low-calorie items on your plate first. Start with the salad, soup and veggies. By the time you get to the chicken and starches you will hopefully be full enough to be content with smaller portions of the higher-calorie choices.

Finally, some dieticians advise their dieting clients not to eat out. That's right. They believe eating at home is safer. But our thought is you have to eat out eventually so why not learn how while your resolve is high?

When you're on a diet, eating in a restaurant can be a challenge, because most restaurant portions are huge, and can easily total more than 1,000 Calories. When eating in a restaurant decide how much to eat – and take the remainder home. A good general rule of thumb is to **eat half and bring the rest home**.

# Day 8 - Recipe

## Baked Salmon with Salsa

This is a simple, straight-forward recipe.  Again, the advantage of a simple recipe is there are no hidden calories.

    4  5 oz salmon fillets
    6  Tbsp bottled tomato-pepper salsa

Brown salmon fillets in non-stick pan and place in baking dish.  Put fillets in an oven preheated to 350 °F for about 10 minutes.  Plate the salmon. Stir prepared tomato-pepper salsa and spoon it over the salmon.

**Serves 4**.  One salmon fillet is about 215 Calories.

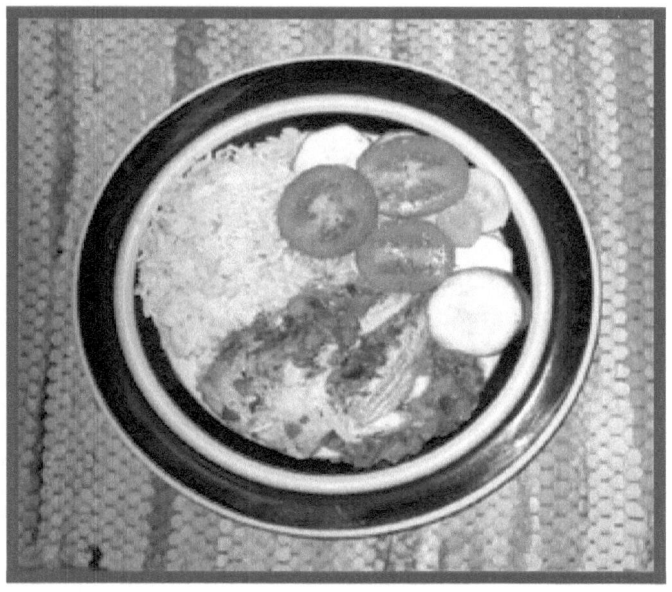

# Day 9 - Recipe

## Veggie Burger

Vegetable-based burgers can be purchased at your local supermarket. The patty of a veggie burger can be made from vegetables, soy, nuts, mushrooms, textured vegetable protein, dairy, or a combination of these foods.

Two popular veggie burgers are the Boca Burger and Gardenburger. The Boca Burger is made chiefly from soy protein and wheat gluten. (Boca Burger patties are 2.5 oz each and range from 60 to 90 Calories.) The original Gardenburger is made from mushrooms, onions, brown rice, rolled oats, cheese, and spices. (Gardenburger patties are 2.5 oz each and about 100 Calories.)

To prepare, follow package directions. The version shown below has an added slice of low-fat cheddar cheese. The lettuce, tomato and ketchup shown actually add very few extra calories.

The veggie burger patty plus low-fat cheese amounts to approximately 150 Calories. Add a seeded roll and the total rises to 290 Calories.

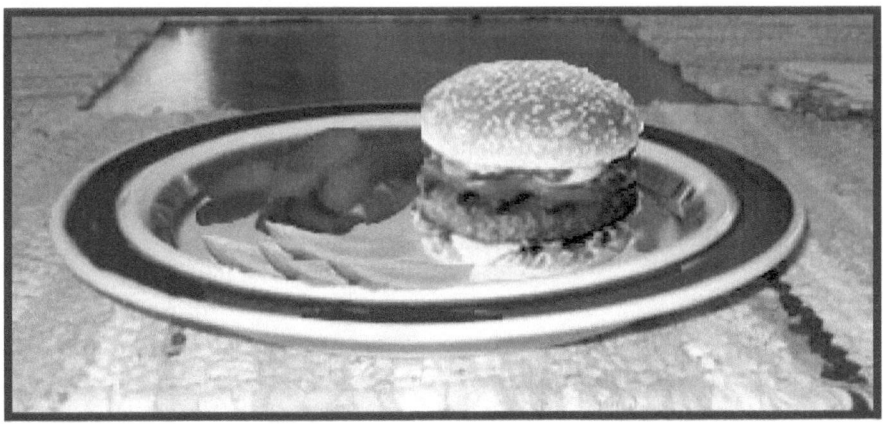

# Day 10 - Recipe

## <u>Wild Blueberry Pancakes</u>

This recipe makes a relatively low calorie, wholesome batch of delicious wild blueberry-whole wheat-buttermilk pancakes.

   1 cup whole-wheat flour
   1 cup buttermilk
   1 egg
   1 Tbsp vegetable oil
   1 tsp baking powder
   ½ tsp baking soda

Stir ingredients until blended. Add ¾ cup blueberries and gently stir. Using medium heat, preheat a non-stick skillet coated with cooking spray. Pour slightly less than ¼ cup of batter onto skillet per pancake. Cook slowly until bubbles break on surface of pancake. Turn and cook until other side is lightly browned. Makes 8 pancakes.

Pictured below are wild-blueberry pancakes with two slices of turkey bacon.

<u>Serves 4</u>. Each pancake is about 95 Calories

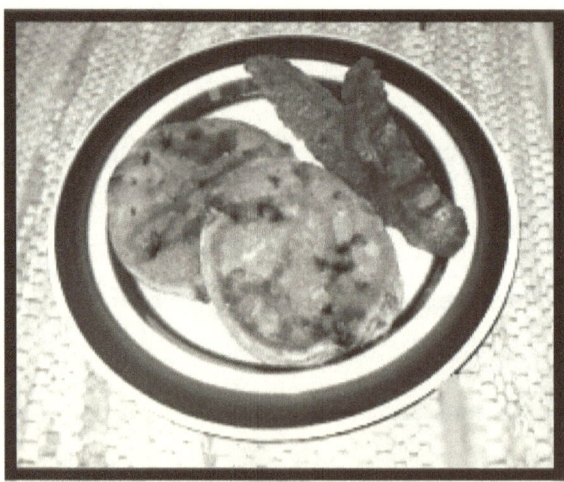

# NoPaperPress eBooks and Paperbacks

100-Day Super Diet-1200 Cal*
100-Day Super Diet-1500 Cal*
100-Day No-Cooking Diet-1200 Cal*
100-Day No-Cooking Diet-1500 Cal*
90-Day Smart Diet-1200 Cal*
90-Day Smart Diet-1500 Cal*
90-Day No-Cooking Diet - 1200 Cal*
90-Day No-Cooking Diet - 1500 Cal*
90-Day Perfect Diet - 1200 Cal*
90-Day Perfect Diet - 1500 Cal*
60-Day Perfect Diet-1200 Cal*
60-Day Perfect Diet-1500 Cal*
50-Day Flex Diet-1200 Cal*
50-Day Flex Diet-1500 Cal*
30-Day Quick Diet - Women*
30-Day Quick Diet for Men*
30-Day No-Cooking Diet*
30-Day Diet for Women - Metric*
30-Day Diet for Men - Metric*
25 Day Easy Diet-1200 Cal*
25 Day Easy Diet-1500 Cal*
25-Day No-Cooking Diet
10-Day Express Diet
10-Day No-Cooking Diet*
7-Day Diet for Women*
7-Day Diet for Men*
7-Day No-Cooking Diets*
90-Day Gluten-Free Diet-1200 Cal*
90-Day Gluten-Free Diet-1500 Cal*
30-Day Gluten-Free Quick Diet*
30-Day Gluten-Free No-Cooking Diet*
7-Day Diet for Women - Metric*
7-Day Diet for Men - Metric
7-Day Gluten-Free Express Diet*
7-Day Gluten-Free No-Cooking Diet*
90-Day Vegetarian Diet-1200 Cal*
90-Day Vegetarian Diet-1500 Cal*
30-Day Vegetarian Diet*
7-Day Vegetarian Diet*
Weight Loss for Women*
Weight Loss for Women - Metric
Weight Loss for Women - UK
Weight Loss for Men*
Maximum Weight Loss - 1200 Cal*
Maximum Weight Loss - 1500 Cal*

Weight Loss for Men - Metric*
Maximum Weight Loss- 1200 Cal*
Maximum Weight Loss- 1500 Cal*
Weight Control - U.S. Edition*
Weight Control - Metric. Edition
Professional Weight Control Women - U.S.
Professional Weight Control Women - Metric
Professional Weight Control Men - U.S.
Professional Weight Control Men - Metric
Weight Maintenance - U.S. Ed*
Weight Maintenance - Metric. Ed*
Weight Maintenance - UK Ed
Weight Loss for Senior Men*
Weight Loss for Senior Women*
Eat Smart - U.S. Edition*
Eat Smart - Metric Edition
30-Day Mediterranean Diet
Exercise Smart - U.S. Edition*
Exercise Smart - Metric Edition
Exercise Smart - UK Edition*
Total Fitness - U.S. Edition
Total Fitness - Metric Edition
Total Fitness - UK Edition
Total Fitness for Women-U.S. Ed*
Total Fitness for Women - Metric
Total Fitness for Women - UK Ed
Total Fitness for Men - U.S. Ed*
Total Fitness for Men- Metric Ed*
Total Fitness for Men - UK Ed
Senior Fitness - U.S. Edition*
Senior Fitness - Metric Edition*
Senior Fitness - UK Edition*
Computer Diet - U.S. Edition*
Computer Diet - Metric Ed*
Reliable Weight Loss - U.S. Ed
101 Weight Loss Tips*
101 Healthy Eating Tips*
101 Lifelong Fitness Tips*
101 Weight Maintenance Tips
101 Weight Loss Recipes
101 GF Weight Loss Recipes
101 Veggie Weight Loss Recipes*
30-Day Mediterranean Diet*
90-Day Mediterranean Diet - 1200 Cal*
90-Day Mediterranean Diet - 1500 Cal*

* These titles are available as both ebooks and paperbacks. Our ebooks are sold by Amazon, Apple, Google, Barnes & Noble and Kobo, but our paperbacks are only sold by Amazon.

**Vincent W. Antonetti**, Ph.D. is a professor emeritus at Manhattan College. He is a weight control and fitness expert who has lectured on fitness at IBM 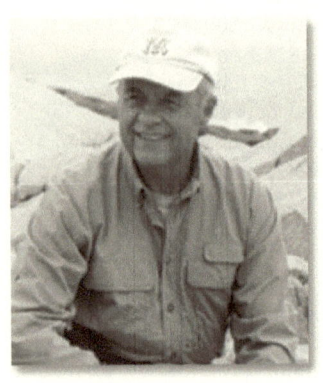 Management and Professional Development classes and often speaks on fitness and weight control. Among his many publications is his highly regarded "The Equations Governing Weight Change in Human Beings," published in the prestigious American Journal of Clinical Nutrition. This paper was the first to develop an accurate equation to calculate weight loss. Dr. Antonetti's critically acclaimed book The Computer Diet was given Consumer Guide magazine's highest recommendation. Recently, Dr. Antonetti coauthored "A Computational Tool to Simulate Energy Balance Components in Pharmacological Interventions," presented at Obesity Week 2016. He also co-authored (with Professor Diana Thomas) "Dynamic Modeling of Energy Expenditure to Estimate Dietary Energy Intake," Chapter 12 in Advances in the Assessment of Dietary Intake, published July 2017 by CRC Press. He is the author of 80 books (ebooks and paperbacks), all concerning weight control, fitness and nutrition. Most of Dr. Antonetti's books are listed at: www.nopaperpress.com.

Professor Antonetti is a life long exercise and nutrition enthusiast. Although a senior citizen he still maintains a vigorous physical fitness program - and has managed to maintain his weight to within 2 lbs of the 154 lbs it was when he graduated from college many years ago. He is semi-retired and lives in The Villages, Florida.

# Disclaimer

This book offers general weight control, exercise and nutrition information. It is not a medical manual and the author does not claim to be medically qualified. The material in this book is not intended to be a substitute for medical counseling. Everyone should have a medical checkup before beginning a weight maintenance program. Moreover, the physician conducting the medical exam should be made aware of and should approve the specific weight control program planned. Additionally, while the author and publisher have made every effort to ensure the accuracy of the information in this book, they make no representations or warranties regarding its accuracy or completeness. Further, neither the author nor publisher assume liability for any medical problems that might result from applying the methods in this book, or for any loss of profit, or any other commercial damages, including but not limited to special, incidental, consequential or other damages, and any such liability is hereby expressly disclaimed.